The

Program 120®

Preventive Medicine

Patient Handbook B

FOR

FEMALES

(Chapter 11 Modern HRT)

Steps We Use To Enhance Healing Through Our Human Bodies' Physiological Mechanisms

On Hormone Replacement Therapy

The members of the media, including even some more educated in the medical media, usually report incorrectly on hormones and hormone replacement therapy showing their ignorance and inappropriate bias. This has in turn misinformed physicians who are to trusting and uninformed – maybe even your physician was this way at one time. Horse hormones (i.e. conjugated equine estrogens or CEE) and synthetic hormones such as medroxyprogesterone and injectable anabolic steroids) ARE NOT human hormones. Human hormones, we believe, are safe when given in the proper milieu and amounts and the literature clearly supports this. These biologically identical human hormones (i.e. bio-identical hormones) are a critical part of unbiased and true preventive medicine program and here we lay out our case.

Thank you for your consideration of these critical issues…

Modern Hormone Replacement Therapy

Paradigm Shift

Throughout this text we've included data on viable hormone options for prevention of deadly diseases – they've been included because they're in the literature and because they work. Now we need to take this debate to the next level, one again supported in the literature, but one that will still require you to undergo a serious paradigm shift in the way you think and view patients and their lab results. We and our patients were in our hormonal prime in our 20s and ideally we should try to optimize hormone levels back to this period. *There is not one study in the literature that disagrees with this premise* but there are a huge number of studies that not only agree with this premise but use these same optimized numbers as parameters in their studies.

Optimization examples in the literature

Example 1

This is not the usual testosterone lab norm for older patients as reflected in this study – they use the same optimized values for 20-somethings that we suggest because these are ideal.

Fukui M, Kitagawa Y, Nakamura N, Kadono M, Mogami S, Hirata C, Ichio N, Wada K, Hasegawa G, Yoshikawa T. **Association between serum testosterone concentration and carotid atherosclerosis in men with type 2 diabetes**. *Diabetes Care*. 2003 Jun;26(6):1869-73.

They conclude – "serum F-tes [free testosterone] concentration is inversely associated with carotid atherosclerosis determined by ultrasonographically evaluated IMT and PS in men with type 2 diabetes." Their lab values (by their lab ranges) Serum free and T-tes concentrations (normal ranges 14.0–40.0 pg/ml and 2.7–10.7 ng/ml, respectively).

Example 2

First, this is not the usual lab norm for 60 year old plus patients as reflected in this study – they use the same IGF-1 values we suggest today derived from 20-somethings because these are ideal. Second, this is THE landmark article by Daniel Rudman that started the "anti-aging" medicine movement in the USA and was published in THE peer reviewed journal here in the USA.

Rudman D, Feller AG, Nagraj HS, Gergans GA, Lalitha PY, Goldberg AF, Schlenker RA, Cohn L, Rudman IW, Mattson DE. **Effects of human growth hormone in men over 60 years old**. *N Engl J Med*. 1990 Jul 5;323(1):1-6.

After referring to their optimized levels they then [rightly] conclude – "diminished secretion of growth hormone is responsible in part for the decrease of lean body mass, the expansion of adipose-tissue mass, and the thinning of the skin that occur in old age."

Clearly this shows that major studies published in peer review journals use optimal lab levels of a younger ideal populations but what do experts in various fields think about this level optimization?

Example 3

In his landmark article and review entitled **Menopause** published in the *Medical Clinics of North America* in November of 1995, Joel Hargrove M.D. who was director of the menopause clinics in the Department of Obstetrics and Gynecology, Vanderbilt University School of Medicine, in Nashville, Tennessee, not only refers to optimizing estrogen (50-150 pg/ml) and DHEA levels (800-3300 ng/ml) but advises using human biologically identical versions when giving HRT. This is a great article that we would advise any physician who's interested in finding and copying for an excellent future reference.

Experts opine about optimization

Example 1
J Gerontol A Biol Sci Med Sci. 1999 Mar;54(3):M111-6.
Thyroid hormones: positive relationships with cognition in healthy, euthyroid older men.
Prinz PN, Scanlan JM, Vitaliano PP, Moe KE, Borson S, Toivola B, Merriam GR, Larsen LH, Reed HL.

What was said – "Our data suggest that older subjects require circulating thyroid hormones in *middle to high levels* in order to maintain optimal brain functioning." *[Not age related norms but the optimized levels we are currently suggesting plus they gave T3 with the T4.]*

Example 2
Infertility and Reproductive Clinics of North America
An Alternative Method of Hormone Replacement Therapy using the Natural Sex Steroids
Joel T. Hargrove, MD, and Kevin G. Osteen, PhD.

What was said – "Because the normal menstrual cycle is characterized by *estradiol levels ranging from 50-150 pg/ml* of serum, we believe these values are reasonable as guidelines for determining replacement of estradiol." *[Again, not age related norms but the optimized levels we suggest plus they advise giving bio-identical hormones.]*

Example 3
Cortlandt Forum, pp 392-394, July 2000.
Clinical Update. Menopause Management, Part 1: Perimenopausal Transition and Early Menopause.
Regula Burki, MD, Clinical Instructor at the University of Utah School of Medicine

What she said – "Estrogen replacement will stop hot flashes but may require *higher than physiologic premenopausal levels.*"

From these statements and studies (and all the others out there) it should be easy to conclude that we, as regular practitioners in the medical community, should not only prescribe bio-identical human hormones, which clearly make patients feel much better by improving their quality of life *[In the end what else are we, as medical practitioners, here for?]*, but measure these patient's subsequent serum levels based on these optimized lab levels.

What Lab Norms Mean

Lab norms are determined by what at least 1000 average patients of that particular age group had measured over the previous 5-10 years. These are not optimized levels – these are just norms for that age group (which will always be too low). For optimized levels compare to patients who are about 28 years of age.

The Hormonal or Neuroendocrine Theory of Aging

Basically first proposed by Professor Vladimir Dilman and Ward Dean MD, the hormonal theory elaborates on aging by focusing on the neuroendocrine system. This system is a network of biochemicals that govern the release of hormones which are altered by the gland called the *hypothalamus* located in the brain. The hypothalamus controls various feedback mechanisms to instruct other organs and glands to release their hormones. The hypothalamus, acting as a master gland, also responds to the body hormone levels as a guide to the overall hormonal activity. As we grow older the hypothalamus loses its precision regulatory ability and the receptors which uptake individual hormones become less sensitive to them (thyroid receptors in the periphery for example[1]). Accordingly, as we age the secretion of many hormones declines and their effectiveness (compared unit to unit) is also reduced due to the receptors becoming less functional.

One theory for the hypothalamus loss of regulation is that it is damaged by the hormone *cortisol*. Cortisol is produced from the *adrenal glands* (located on the kidneys) and cortisol is considered to be a dark-hormone responsible for stress. It is known to be one of the few hormones that increase with age. As discussed in other chapters in this book, the effects of cortisol floating around in your body can be offset by nutriceutically available hormones such as melatonin.

If cortisol damages the hypothalamus, then over time this becomes a vicious cycle of continued hypothalamic damage, leading to an ever increasing degree of cortisol production and thus more hypothalamic damage. A catch-22 situation ensues.

This damage could then lead to hormonal imbalance as the hypothalamus loses its ability to control the system. Such an argument demands the use of cortisol *adjusters* (such as DHEA, or Phenytoin) to help slow down the cortisol accumulation. The decline in the functional capability if peripheral receptors can be partially offset by receptor resensitizers such as the drug Metformin (which improves insulin sensitivity).

So to prevent aging, to keep us in that young healthy rich hormonal milieu where we had so much fun *and optimal health*, we need hormones that are biologically identical to those we humans produce in our own bodies and in the proper amounts that are reflected in the levels we lived with while we were in our prime (age 25-32). As we've illustrated already the literature is replete with studies and articles in support of these positions.

Key HRT Studies That Wrongly Ruined HRT For Everybody

HERS (Heart and Estrogen/progestin Replacement Study[2]): Participants were postmenopausal women with previously diagnosed CHD who were randomly assigned to receive conjugated equine estrogens and medroxyprogesterone or identical placebo and then followed-up for an average of 4.1 years. The conclusion was that hormone therapy had no overall effect on CHD risk in the HERS trial despite the expected favorable effects on HDL-C and LDL-C levels. The real outcome though has been the systematic horrification of millions of women and their physicians worldwide and their scaring away from using or taking any female hormones — synthetic side effect intensive hormones being erroneously discussed in the popular and medical press as if they were real human hormones.

For example, the HERS study as reported by Denise Grady in the February 6, 2001 edition of *The New York Times* in her article titled **A New Look At Estrogen And Stroke**, she discusses the study as reported in *Circulation* and concluded that women with heart disease cannot assume hormone replacement therapy will protect them from stroke. In her explanation she did not differentiate between the synthetic progestational agent/equine conjugated estrones combination used in the study and real-for goodness human hormones that were available then and are still (see the 1995 article **Menopause** in *The Medical Clinics of North America* by Joel Hargrove). From this and other articles comes the fear we face today when we mention HRT.

WHI (Women's Health Initiative Postmenopausal Hormone Therapy Trials[3]) This is the study that we've all heard so much about. Created by the National Institutes of Health (NIH) -- specifically, the National Heart, Lung and Blood Institute (NHLBI) this study was designed to define the risks and benefits of interventions, notably hormone therapy, to potentially prevent heart disease, breast and colorectal cancer, and osteoporotic fractures in postmenopausal women, on the basis of results from this study and their interpretation by the lead investigators, "guidelines for the use of hormone therapy in postmenopausal women changed. For the study as a whole…161,809 women aged 50 to 79 years were enrolled in either an observational study or clinical trials of low dietary fat vs. self-selected diet, estrogen and progesterone therapy (HT) or estrogen therapy alone (ET) vs. placebo, or calcium and vitamin D supplementation vs. placebo."

Wait…

Huh? What? This study used estrogen and progesterone? Really?

Naah, not really! Read on…

"The larger of the 2 studies evaluating postmenopausal hormone therapy randomized nonhysterectomized women to estrogen plus progestin (0.625 mg conjugated equine estrogens [CEE] + 2.5 mg medroxyprogesterone acetate (MPA), *Prempro®*, N = 8506 women) or placebo (N = 8102 women). Monitoring of these subjects began in the fall of 1997 and was scheduled to last until 2005. However, the Data Safety Monitoring Board (DSMB) terminated the HT arm of the WHI early when a predetermined threshold of excess cases of breast cancer was reached.[4] The smaller hormone study involved 10,739 women who had undergone hysterectomy; they were randomized to receive estrogen alone (0.625 CEE, *Premarin®*) or placebo. The ET arm was terminated March 2, 2004 -- also early -- because of increased risk of stroke."

MEDROXYPROGESTERONE and CONJUGATED EQUINE ESTRONES are NOT human hormones! Human serum medroxyprogesterone levels are not even measurable! And they exposed 161,809 women to this FDA approved big money-making patented drug?

Let's see what the press had to say – surely they caught this slip…

As reported by Leslie Berger in the June 6, 2004 edition of *The New York Times* in her article titled **TWO YEARS AFTER; On Hormone Therapy, the Dust Is Still Settling** where she notes that two years after the bombshell results of the WHI was dropped on hormone replacement therapy, there were at that time signs that the rush away from the drugs was finally ending. She then goes onto note that how in July 2002, a federal study, part of the Women's Health Initiative, was halted when its data showed the dangers of hormone therapy outweighing its long-term benefits. After the study sales of the drugs -- estrogen and estrogen-progestin – had plunged.

Well, it's a little better – they called it progestin this time but still did not mention human hormones nor did they really differentiate between progestins (synthetics) and progesterone (human hormone).

Or how about the recent study on HRT and breast cancer? The Million Women Study?

Look at the abstract in Pub Med by Reeves GK, et al. (**For the Million Women Study Collaborators. Cancer Research UK Epidemiology Unit, University of Oxford, UK.** *Hormonal therapy for menopause and breast-cancer risk by histological type: a cohort study and meta-analysis.* **Lancet Oncol. 2006 Nov;7(11):910-8.**). There is no mention in this abstract (we presume is written by health care professionals) as to what kind of hormones which were actually used (synthetics and non-human hormones: equine conjugated estrogens and progestogens) and you as a professional are left assuming all hormone replacement therapies are going to cause some level of breast cancer, when the literature is replete with completely opposite observations.

History Questions – Start Here Before They Even See You

Female Hormonal History Questions

1. Are you concerned about facial skin wrinkles? Other skin wrinkles?
2. Are you concerned about depression? Do you ever feel blue?
3. Are you concerned about improving your sex life?
4. Are you concerned about keeping strong?
5. Are you concerned about keeping fit?
6. Are you concerned about healthy bones?
7. Have you ever been told you have osteoporosis?
8. Any family history of osteoporosis?
9. Have you been through menopause?
10. When did your other go through menopause?
11. What are your periods like?
12. How many pregnancies have you had? How many deliveries?
13. Do you ever have sexual problems?
14. Every have difficulty getting sexually aroused?
15. Ever feel breathlessness?
16. Are you concerned about memory loss?
17. Do you ever lose your way while driving or shopping?
18. Are you concerned about increased weight?
19. Have you gained weight lately or in the last few years? If so, how much?
20. Are you concerned about decreased libido (decreased sex drive)?
21. Are you concerned about dry eyes, or dry skin, or a dry vagina?
22. Are you concerned about tooth loss?
23. Do you ever feel fatigue?
24. Are you concerned about your genitalia drying and shriveling up?
25. Are you concerned about reducing your risk of heart disease?
26. Do you drink alcohol? How much?
27. Do you take narcotics? How often? Which ones?
28. Have you had painful joints or been diagnosed with osteoarthritis?
29. Have you ever had breast, ovarian or uterine/cervical cancer?

Male Hormonal History Questions

1. Are you concerned about facial skin wrinkles? Other skin wrinkles?
2. Are you concerned about depression? Do you ever feel blue?
3. Are you concerned about improving your sex life?
4. Are you concerned about keeping strong?
5. Are you concerned about keeping fit?
6. Have your muscles gotten smaller lately or in recent years?
7. Are you concerned about healthy bones?
8. Have you ever been told you have osteoporosis?
9. Any family history of male osteoporosis?
10. Have you been through "male menopause?"
11. When did your father go through "male menopause?"
12. Do you ever have sexual problems?
13. Every have difficulty getting sexually aroused?
14. Do you have trouble maintaining an erection once you are aroused?
15. Do your ejaculations seem normal?
16. Ever feel breathlessness (shortness of breath) while having sex?
17. Ever feel breathlessness at all?
18. Do you exercise?
19. Has your endurance decreased, stayed about the same, or improved?
20. Are you concerned about memory loss?
21. Do you ever lose your way while driving or shopping?

22. Are you concerned about increased weight?
23. Have you gained weight lately or in the last few years? If so, how much?
24. Are you concerned about decreased libido (decreased sex drive)?
25. Do you ever feel fatigue?
26. Are you concerned about reducing your risk of heart disease?
27. Do you drink alcohol? How much?
28. Do you take narcotics? How often? Which ones?
29. Have you ever had prostate, breast, or testicular cancer?

Powerful Hormonal Options

For years we thought patented non-bio-identical hormones were the best way – subsequently we've now found that HRT with biologically identical human hormones is more natural and more beneficial than almost anything else

Rules of This Handbook

From now on all hormones discussed as to be prescribed are compounded hormones that are biologically identical to human hormones. This text is driven by the facts and the research, NOT by pharmaceutical companies. This is absolutely critical, because there are no side effects in any age group which have ever been reported with these exact human hormones when they are given properly and in the correct dose and milieu (please report if you find such a study to our website). To buttress our point, levels are tracked with the same exact serum blood tests that you use to track endogenous hormones (try doing that with the medroxyprogesterone in Provera®).

These ARE true human hormones.

A. Pregnenolone

Pregnenolone, actually usually available as an OTC nutriceutical, is another master hormone or prohormone similar in many ways to DHEA (see below). Most critically pregnenolone seems to give neuroprotection and cognitive protection. Notable that pregnenolone is the major steroid precursor in humans[4]. It is also a "neurosteroid" and possesses intrinsic behavioral and brain effects in animals, affecting the GABA(A) and other receptors.

Pregnenolone Summary

1. Pregnenolone is THE major steroid and neurosteroid precursor[5].
2. Pregnenolone is neuroprotective and promotes cellular repair in the brain[6].
3. Pregnenolone is a potent memory enhancer especially in those with brain injuries and the elderly[7].
4. Pregnenolone helps with traumatic brain and spinal chord injury recovery and healing[8].
5. Pregnenolone improves rheumatoid arthritis and the pain associated with RA[9].
6. Pregnenolone helps Alzheimer's disease[10] [11].
7. Pregnenolone has no side effects.
8. Pregnenolone should be taken preventatively before symptoms appear.

Pregnenolone Practice Gems

1. Every patient >40 years of age should receive this.
2. Every patient with a TBI (traumatic brain injury) should receive this!
3. Dose is 100 mgm every day for males and females.
4. There is no reason to check the level because there's no side effect and no overdosing.

B. Melatonin

Melatonin is a natural neurotransmitter-like hormone produced primarily by the pineal gland and does many beneficial things for the human body.

The best recent review of melatonin can be found in Medscape in the MedGenMed Neurology & Neurosurgery section entitled "The Therapeutic Potential of Melatonin: A Review of the Science [12].

Here are just a few **benefits of melatonin**:

1. Appropriate for people 35 and older[13]. Very safe with no known side effects or overdose potential.

2. One of the strongest available natural endogenous antioxidant[14].
   A. Protects and heals brain damage from trauma (stroke or TBI)[15].
   B. Anti-inflammatory at the endothelium of the blood vessels[16].
   C. Prevents migraine headaches[17].
   D. Treats cluster headaches[18].
   E. Not only prevents but treats lung cancer[19].
   F. Most importantly it replenishes your glutathione level which is a hormonal anti-oxidant that protects against cardiovascular disease, (this glutathione especially occurs in diabetic patients[20] where melatonin should almost always be given).
   G. Protects against cataracts[21] (this is HUGE! How many elderly patients do you have with cataracts?).
   H. Efficient for the treatment of major depressive disorder and bipolar affective disorder[22].
   I. Lowers cholesterol[23].
   J. Cardioprotective through anti-oxidant activity[24].
   K. Alleviates some of the worst symptoms of sundowning[25] (the early nocturnal confusion and increased activity of Alzheimer's patients) but has recently been shown to help prevent the worsening dementia of Alzheimer's disease[26]!
   L. Improves Sleep Disturbances[27]
   M. Reduces Jet Lag[28]
   N. Reduces Insomnia[29]
   O. Treats Narcolepsy[30]
   P. Improves Endocrine Function and Immunity[31]
   Q. Reduces Risk of Breast Cancer[32]
   R. Reduces Risk of Prostate Cancer[33] [34]
   S. Reduces Risk of Colon Cancer[35] [36]
   T. Reduces Essential Hypertension in men and women[37] -- the BEST benefit.
   U. Decreases Nocturia[38] and Renal Disease (reduces interstitial inflammation of the kidneys[39]) – this is another GREAT benefit.
   V. Acts as a Powerful Antioxidant[40]
   X. Increases expression of the antioxidant enzymes superoxide dismutase and glutathione peroxidase[41].

5. Melatonin administration leads to increased expression of the very potent antioxidant enzymes superoxide dismutase and glutathione peroxidase[42].

6. Cools the endothelium, reduces dreaded silent inflammation[43].

7. In men, when taken at night, can (at least partially) lower essential hypertension alone[44]! Works in women[45], also.

8. Melatonin 20 mgm at night is THE only drug/med/hormone that will increase a patient's (undergoing chemotherapy or suffering from ITP[46]) platelet/thrombocyte count[47]! Remember this – this is a key trick to use if one your patient develops a low platelet count!

9. You can now get an agonist form of melatonin as a prescription – Ramelteon (Rozerem®) which is 8 mgm of a highly selective melatonin receptor Type 1 and 2 agonist[48]. It is also the only sleep aid not scheduled (so it's not considered habituating) under DEA law.

10. Take micronized sustained release at night to help sleep[49].

    a. 10% of patients will have no sleep effect – increase dose slowly ever few days until they get groggy the next AM then cut back a dose(1-30 mgm total)
    b. 1% will have adverse effect -- stop it or give very low dose.
    c. Tends to change hair color back to normal (from gray etc) no matter how old.
    d. Take 1 hour prior to bed.
    e. Titrate up slowly; it's really just trial and error. Average male dose is 9-40 mgm for men less for women. **Maximum dose** is 45 mgm each night.
    f. Nightmares that don't stop may require you change the type of melatonin.

C. Thymus

The thymus gland is located behind the sternum and is very large at birth but essentially disappears by the time we get to 40-50 years of age. It is vital in providing immunity to our bodies. Thymic peptides nurture T-cells as they mature into CD4 and CD8 cells[50]. CD4 cells are also known as helper cells because they recognize foreign objects and help guide CD8 killer cells and antibodies to those objects. T-Lymphocytes are derived from the thymus while B-lymphocytes are derived from the bone marrow. T-lymphocyte cells fight viral infections while B-cells fight bacterial infections, so the thymus us critical in HIV, herpes and other viral infections.

It has been theorized in the past that thymic peptide replacement could replenish the immunities missing due to the aging atrophy of the thymus. Thymic Protein A, which activates the T-4 helper cell (CD4 T-lymphocyte) and was the first of these native biologically active proteins to become commercially available (can be taken sublingually) made by a company called ProBoost™.

A number of nutrients, trace elements, and vitamins (e.g., zinc, selenium, copper, vitamins A, D, and E) are also critical to hematopoiesis. Zinc seems to be the best studied and well known nutrient associated with active T-cell function.

But if your thymus is hypofunctional (because of age or disease) and you are having problems with viral infections (shingles, herpes, HIV[51]) then a drug called ProBoost Thymic Protein A® may be beneficial. It has been shown to dramatically boost CD4 cell activity and this leads to a sometimes dramatic increase in your antiviral capabilities. This is a thymic hormone, the only one to date that increases CD4 activity. And is well worth looking into (though it is unclear at press time why they are a food nutriceutical and not FDA approved for insurance coverage) but the price seems reasonable.

This could cover: **Epstein Barr (EBV or Mononucleoosis)**

Hepatitis B, C and others

HIV

Herpes Zoster or Shingles

This appears to work especially well in the elderly. So if you have a patient or loved one with shingles or hepatitis C this might be a significant option and currently the only legitimate way to boost your thymus and antiviral activity.

Thymus Summary and Practice Gems

Make sure all your micronutrients are in place – especially zinc.

As we age, and if we develop a viral problem (such as shingles), then consider **ProBoost Thymic Protein A®** to boost your T-Cell function.

Also for your homosexual or sexually active patients it may not be a bad idea.

D. DHEA (Dehydroepiandrosterone)

DHEA is produced in the brain but more so in the adrenal cortex and is a precursor to testosterone, estrogen, and progesterone, plus acts as a neurotransmitter[52]. DHEA is secreted almost exclusively by the adrenal glands[53]. In human males, 5-30% of circulating DHEA is secreted by testes, and in women, the adrenals are the primary source. Converted to its sulfated form (DHEAS) in peripheral and adrenal tissues, it has only limited hormonal potency. The primary form in circulation is DHEAS, which is present in higher concentrations than DHEA in human serum[54].

Dehydroepiandrosterone (DHEA) therapy, currently an OTC nutriceutical, is a little controversial due to sensationalized reports of epidemiologic studies and the over-the-counter availability of DHEA. DHEA is unique compared with other adrenal steroids because of the fluctuation in serum levels found from birth into advancing age but the lower endogenous levels of DHEA and DHEA sulfate found in advancing age have been correlated with a myriad of health conditions[55].

Increases Serum Androgen Levels

Clinical trials suggest that at least 50mg of oral DHEA can increase serum androgen levels to within the physiologic range for adults with primary and secondary adrenal insufficiency, possibly improve sexual function, improve mood and self-esteem, and decrease fatigue and exhaustion[56]. This is because DHEA acts as a prohormone increasing the levels of androgens such as androstenedione and testosterone[57]. In non-technical terms maintaining physiologic levels of DHEA can "load the gun" in patients who are pro-hormone exhausted increasing testosterone levels in females and allowing adequate production in males who have the right supportive characteristics in place to create testosterone. *[Note these studies may support 50 mgm but read below for more realistic real life doses of 0.5-75 mgm.]*

Endogenous Production Declines With Age

Human DHEA and DHEA-S levels decline linearly and systematically with age and suggest the potential importance of that parameter as a biomarker of ageing[58].

Dosing

Give a sustained release pharmaceutical grade capsule. Study after study give much higher doses than these while pushing levels well beyond these, so don't be afraid optimize your doses and levels to get maximum benefits[59]. Men should take 50 mgm every AM and if weight is > 200 lbs give them 100 mgm every morning.

Males	**Dose**
Every man > 40 years of age	5-100 mgm daily
(Weight >200 lbs?)	Closer to 100 mgm daily
	(Some may require as little as
	10 mgm per day, so reduce the dose.)

Females	Dose
Postmenopausal & < 50 years old	10-15 mgm a day
Postmenopausal & >50 years old	10-25 mgm a day

Levels (Measured as DHEAS)

Before Treatment	DHEAS LEVEL
Postmenopausal/ Postandropausal	50-140 µg/dL

Optimized

Males	500-660 µg/dL
Females	200-250 µg/dL

Benefits

Optimized levels protect against and/or help reduce:

1. Arteriosclerosis (prevents lipid peroxidation)[60].
2. Vasculopathy of coronary allografts (protects post-CABG patients)[61].
3. Death from ANY form of cardiovascular disease (according to the New England Journal of Medicine a low level of DHEA in a man over 50 is an independent risk factor[62] -- peer reviewed greatest journal in the USA ever where when they increased levels 100 µg/dL above the study levels of 140 µg/dL there was a 36% reduction in mortality from *any* cause and a 48% reduction in CVD causes. What more can we say? Do NOT let your patients go untreated!)
4. Conditions associated with insulin resistance and hyperinsulinemia, such as obesity, hypertension, and untreated Type 2 Diabetes.[63]
5. Visceral obesity[64].
6. Autoimmune diseases such as SLE[65], Herpes, Epstein-Barr (boosts immune system), and even HIV[66].
7. Erectile dysfunction[67].
8. Osteoporosis in women and men[68].
9. Low levels of DHEA and DHEAS are factors in increasing obesity and adiposity[69].

Optimized DHEA levels cause:
1. Improved energy levels[70].
2. Improved mood and well being and quality of life[71].
3. Improvement of depression[72].
4. Increased testosterone, progesterone, and estrogen levels downstream in the human body – hormones beneficial in the protection against CVD (avoid the Keto-7 version some pharmacists compound or you will not get these "downstream" hormonal benefits).
5. Improved insulin sensitivity, reduced diabetes symptoms and effects[73].
6. Increased abdominal fat weight loss (reducing diabetes risks)[74].
7. Improved memory[75].
8. Improved psychological well being[76].
9. Boosting of the immune system preventing carcinogenesis[77].
10. The ability to reduce or even replace corticosteroids[78].
11. Significantly enhances bone mineral density (BMD)[79].
12. Elevates IGF-1 levels independent of any HGH levels[80].
13. Appears to facilitate wound healing[81] without the adverse effects of estrogen.

Seriously, will a statin do all of this? Will a TZD?

Side Effects of Too Much DHEA

1. Acne – men or women – levels are too high[82], so reduce their dose. Some people are just sensitive to even a little DHEA so don't be afraid to back off the dose a lot. If acne occurs from DHEA you can give Z-Pack® (if they want quicker clearing) and stop DHEA for few days and if they are on 10 mgm a day go to every other day. (Spironolactone would work but would take 6 months.)
2. Hirsutism[83] – occurs in women, usually with darker skin like Asians or Middle Eastern women – DHEAS is too high. Back the dose down.

[Malpractice Warning: Do not give to anyone who's ever had sex hormone responsive cancer (prostate, breast, testicular).]

DHEA Summary

1. DHEA is a prohormone. Biochemically it is the precursor to androstenedione (or "ANDRO") so no need for body builders to take that substance if they have plenty of DHEA on board.
2. Low DHEAS levels at a premenopausal or preandropausal age (or older) indicates markedly increased risk for obesity.
3. Low levels at a premenopausal or preandropausal age (or older) indicates markedly increased risk for insulin resistance and thus Type II Diabetes.
4. Low levels at a premenopausal or preandropausal age (or older) indicates markedly increased risk for hyperlipidemia and thus heart disease or increased stroke risk.
5. Low levels at a premenopausal or preandropausal age (or older) almost always accompanies a markedly increased glucocorticoid level indicating stress (either from age or physical/psychological stress). Remember – low DHEA indicates high cortisol levels!
6. Low levels occur as we get older.
7. The age-related increase in the cortisol/DHEA ratio (secondary to both a decline in DHEA and increase in cortisol) is a *major* determinant of immunological changes observed during aging[84].
8. Low levels at an older age indicate markedly increased risk for depression and cognitive dysfunction or decline. Conversely DHEA improves cognition men[85].
9. DHEA stimulates the immune system and prevents immunosenescence.
10. If you get new acne or peach fuzz (women) on DHEA reduce your dose or stop it.
11. DHEA can help with various rheumatological disorders such as SLE.
12. If you have a patient on prednisone they can reduce or replace their dose by adding DHEA[86].
13. DHEA markedly increases sexual libido and pleasure in postmenopausal women (and maybe postandropausal men).
14. DHEA is an androgenic steroid (thus the acneiform side effects) and will help build muscle.
15. Increasing your DHEA will reduce you cortisol, thus reducing the immune supressance associated with that glucocorticoid.
16. DHEA slows or stops osteoporosis in postmenopausal and premenopausal women[87].
17. DHEA appears to prevent and block the growth of breast cancer[88].
18. Recent studies show adequate DHEA replacement may actually reduce the risk of prostate cancer becoming androgen-independent and thus more aggressive[89].
19. MALPRACTICE WARNING: Have patients sign a release/informed consent if they wish to take and are at high risk for breast cancer or prostate cancer.

E. Thyroid

Thyroid is a great hormone – easy to take with levels that are easy to follow but conversely thyroid hormone supplementation can be controversial and seemingly complicated.

Let's be a little controversial up front – Dr. Purser prefers dessicated animal thyroid – now THAT'S controversial.

Why dessicated animal thyroid?

Because it works and it's inexpensive.

Clearly we have known for many decades that the majority of patients benefit from T4 and T3[90] (for a number of reasons supported by many studies[91] and hard opinions[92] which we detail[93]). Armour Thyroid® is a proven quality product and it contains T4, T3, T2, and T1 and treated levels rise in a clearly controlled and proper manner reflective of appropriate dosing (while the FDA has repeatedly found Synthroid® and the research behind it to be problematic leading to millions of dollars in fines and class action lawsuits[94]). We also believe that measuring and following TSH levels alone are not that helpful and it's clearly best to also follow Free T3 levels[95], since this is the active thyroid hormone at the cellular level, and to optimize those levels as done repeatedly throughout major studies[96] (or you won't get the same results).

Dosing and Manner

Start with 1 grain (60 mgm) a day. For older people start with ¼ or ½ grain a day
Increase at no more than 1 grain per month. Take in the morning (if your patient is taking once per day) on an empty stomach 30 minutes before eating for an optimal result – but always take on an empty stomach[97].

Optimized Levels

Supported in numerous studies (conflicted in others) your patient's Free T3 level should be 3.9 pg/ml or above (if you can -- forget about TSH and T4 levels).

Symptoms of Hypothyroidism and Benefits of Supplementation

What are the **symptoms/sequelae of hypothyroidism** and **benefits of T3/T4 supplementation**?

1. Subclinical hypothyroidism accompanying symptoms may include intolerance to cold, muscle cramps, dry skin, constipation, poor energy levels, fatigue and mental slowness[98].

2. LDL-C was higher in subjects with subclinical hypothyroidism[99].

3. Total cholesterol was higher in subjects with subclinical hypothyroidism[100].

4. Triglycerides were higher in subjects with subclinical hypothyroidism. Supplementing to optimal levels decreases triglyceride levels[101].

5. Supplementing with thyroid decreases total cholesterol and LDL-C[102].

6. Thyroid hormone does not cause weight loss but lends the energy to the patient sufficient for increased exercise that can lead to weight loss.

7. Hypothyroid patients can present with dyspnea on exertion, fatigue, and edema that may be the result of either pericardial effusion or CHF[103].

8. Most patients with CHF have hypothyroidism -- treating CHF with T3 (T3 was given IV in this study) improves cardiac output and vascular resistance[104].

9. Treating with combination therapy (T3 and T4) improves physical and mental well-being (vs. just giving T4), and to accomplish this, the study investigators optimized the serum Free T3 level[105].

10. Experts believe that even mild subclinical hypothyroidism[106] should be treated[107].

11. So-called subclinical hypothyroidism (Low T3 Syndrome for many endocrinologists) patients give many significant changes in a clinical symptom index (the Billewicz scale) in subclinically hypothyroid women (mean age, 50 years) compared with age-matched controls[108].

12. Subclinical hypothyroidism causes elevation in lipoprotein(a) levels increasing atherosclerosis[109]. *[This increases the deadly lipoprotein(a) so it's hard to rationalize why we let this occur when a cheap treatment option like this will clear that up.]*

13. Subclinical hypothyroidism causes significant alterations in memory and mood, including anxiety, depression, and somaticism, all of which return to normal with therapy with T4 AND T3[110].

14. Thyroxine replacement is actually NOT associated with risk of osteoporosis[111].

15. Women with Diffuse hair loss? Try 1-3 grains of thyroid, push the dose a little and after 6 months or so they should have good hair regrowth. Comes out in clumps – very obvious – this is actually a telogen effluvium. Androgenic hair loss is very slow and occurs over a long period of time.

16. Hypothyroidism is associated with breast cancer in post-menopausal women[112]. If they are at some familial risk treat them aggressively.

17. Fibromyalgia can be treated with supraphysiologic doses of thyroid and most of the time you will get good results if not total clearing of the symptoms[113]. This is due to a thyroid hormone resistance[114] or receptor failure so push the dose in these patients (within reason – monitor for potential serious side effects).

18. There is no lab test available to determine thyroid resistance (which appears to be multifactorial in nature) but from an extensive review of the literature receptor problems or even gross failure is much more common than anyone has perceived[115].

19. Synthroid® Rough Conversion Formula: On Synthroid® 0.1 mgm to 1.0 grains (60 mgm) of Armour®.
20. "I tend to treat everybody."[116]

> –David S. Cooper, MD,
> Director of the Division of Endocrinology,
> Sinai Hospital of Baltimore, Maryland.

True Facts On Thyroid

1. Hypothyroidism increases with age[117].
2. The human thyroid system is almost identical to the porcine thyroid system[118].
3. In the human system there are two main thyroid receptors:
   A. Deiodination receptors activate thyroid and convert from T4 to T3 (remember T3 is the active form of thyroid hormone).
   B. Nuclear retinoid receptors for thyroid are on all cells for thyroid hormone to function.
4. Similar to Type 2 Diabetes you can first get thyroid resistance[119] (also termed receptor exhaustion -- first felt to be genetic, we now know this is part of aging[120]) when either the deiodination receptor begins to fail or when the main peripheral retinoid receptors begin to fail[121]. When this happens, thyroid production and levels can rise in the bodies' attempt to overcome this resistance, plus the conversion of T4 to T3 is slowed.
5. According to one article the incidence of the syndromes of resistance to thyroid hormone is *unknown;* a limited survey suggested the occurrence of 1 case in 50,000 live births[122] but by shear

reason and other studies looked at in this chapter we must assume and know that thyroid receptor failure due to aging is *very common*.

6. T3 is the active moiety *at the cellular level* and much less common than T4 in the human body. T4 is inactive and is usually kept in reserve, while T3 is ten times more active and is, by all experts, considered the active thyroid hormone[123].

7. Remember the **symptoms of hypothyroidism**[124]:
    A. Fatigue
    B. Lower then normal body temperature
    C. Greater susceptibility to colds and other viruses (immunospression)
    D. Weight gain
    E. Depression
    F. Dry skin
    G. Headaches
    H. High cholesterol and other hyperlipidemias
    I. Inability of a female to get or maintain a pregnancy[125].

8. Thyroid resistance[126] occurs more often as we get older and is a recognized entity (not a false construct to benefit Armour®). This can be due to a number of reasons but thyroid receptor failure is the most common in the elderly despite many articles to the contrary. The usual cause of this "rare" disorder is felt to be genetic and the gene defect is also tied to insulin receptor failure[127].

9. Other than aging and genetics disorders it is unclear why thyroid receptors fail and thyroid hormone resistance occurs. We would encourage more studies in this area but we suspect as in insulin receptor failure (i.e. insulin resistance) that testosterone and HGH probably assist in maintaining the viability of these receptors.

10. Like in diabetes, thyroid receptor activity, health, and longevity improvement occurs with HGH which also improves end organ resistance. It is broadly believed that giving HGH physiological amounts would be beneficial in thyroid resistance cases or when you suspect someone has failing receptors[128].

11. There are several versions of the deiodinated thyroid hormone beyond the T4 moiety – T3, T2, and T1 -- and all versions come with some activity in peripheral tissues (not just T3) though this activity has not yet been clearly defined in the literature. It is this activity that has led some researchers/practitioners to believe that some patients respond best to desiccated thyroid from the addition of these lesser-known, lesser-understood deiodinated thyroid hormones[129].

12. Because of this reason (#11) and others, dessicated porcine thyroid (Armour® Thyroid) is much preferable to synthetic T3 or T4 in almost all instances.

13. Knoll pharmaceutical who makes Synthroid® falsified some of their data in order to get Synthroid® FDA approved and to be looked on more favorably by the medical community and physicians for some reason keep forgetting this. To support this contention:

"*Company Allegedly Hid Thyroid Research*," Brenda C. Coleman, Associated Press, April 16, 1997. This is where the story broke on Knoll *suppressing* the research allegedly showing that L-thyroxine was *less effective* than the cheaper alternatives (Armour® thyroid or its generics).

We would also refer you to: thyroid.about.com/cs/synthroid1/a/infocenter.htm for details and websites that might inform you more.

Also, from September 1997 -- according to what the FDA had placed in the **Federal register**, "*no currently marketed orally administered levothyroxine sodium product has been shown to demonstrate consistent potency and stability and, thus, no currently marketed orally administered levothyroxine sodium product is generally recognized as safe and effective.*"

14. There was a huge class action lawsuit in the 1990's against Knoll which it settled for an insignificant 87.4 million dollars for this little bit of trickery.

15. The FDA has also told physicians that Armour® is safer and better than Synthroid® but we keep forgetting this. The United States Food and Drug Administration Letter to Synthroid® Manufacturer, Knoll Pharmaceuticals, April 26, 2001 was a scathing response where the FDA

officially denied Knoll's request, meaning that Synthroid had to apply for a new drug application by August of 2001 in order to remain legally on the market.

16. Even the CBS show, **60 MINUTES,** did a news article on television in the late 1990's for the public in regards to Knoll.

17. Armour® is much cheaper than Synthroid®.

18. The four main arguments against using dessicated porcine thyroid (Armour®) are bogus and not supported. We've all heard these. These are:

   A. "The dessicated *bovine* hormone is not even close to human thyroid so why give it?"

   FALSE. The formulation for decades has been PORCINE (pig) thyroid, and NOT bovine (cattle) and it is nearly identical.

   B. "Several years ago, researchers discovered that there was considerable variation in potency from batch to batch of the dessicated thyroid-- in short, a manufacturing quality issue."

   FALSE. Dr. Purser and others before us have looked at this issue extensively, and *have not yet found any research that reported "considerable variation in potency from batch to batch."* But in the August 2001 letter from the FDA (noted above) that Synthroid® was denied because *it* could "not be Generally Recognized as Safe and Effective Because it is of No Fixed Composition."

   C. "Levothyroxine is safer and more potent so why give that weird animal thyroid?"

   FALSE.

   Here we go again. In 1997, the U.S. Food and Drug Administration issued a warning, via the **Federal Register**, that *"no currently marketed orally administered levothyroxine sodium product has been shown to demonstrate consistent potency and stability and, thus, no currently marketed orally administered levothyroxine sodium product is generally recognized as safe and effective."* (**Federal Register**, August 14, 1997)

   D. "Angina or atrial fibrillation occurs more with dessicated thyroid."

   FALSE.

   These symptoms are much more common with excess L-thyroxine[130] (thus the FDA statement above in the **Federal Register**) but more rare with the healthy stew present in Armour® thyroid.

19. Giving the dessicated thyroid to patients allows them the healthy stew or milieu of T4, T3, T2, and T1 floating around in their system and they do have purposes[131]. Almost no doctors can tell you what T1 or T2 do but, they cannot also tell you what they do not do, or if they're even necessary. This is bad. Physicians should give it just to be safe since even the FDA believes dessicated animal thyroid is as or more safe then synthetic levothyroxine (if in doubt, see **Federal Register**, August 14, 1997).

20. The change in lab norms increased the number of Americans with thyroid illness from 13 million to approximately 27 million overnight in 2002! But our clinical experience has told us that even the major laboratories continue to give erroneous "normal ranges" for the tests, simply because they're not aware of the guidelines of the AACE or the information put out by their National Association of Clinical Biochemistry.

21. Now, 48 months after the new directives have been given, doctors are still largely unaware of these new lab guidelines for diagnosis and treatment. NOTICE TO ALL DOCTORS AND THEIR LABS! The TSH range has changed! The FDA also believes dessicated porcine thyroid is better and safer then synthetic T3! (Just in case you forgot again.) Regardless the studies tend to ignore TSH and optimize T4 and T3 levels (the latter mainly because tell us why we should care if the inactive version of the hormone is optimized).

22. General myth on thyroid hormone prescribing (because for this myth it does not matter whether you are prescribing synthetic levothyroxine or dessicated porcine thyroid) goes like this, "Giving too much thyroid will suppress their pituitary and thyroid gland – this is a bad thing." That's right. Not really!

FALSE. It is a bad thing to not give *enough* thyroid hormone but these patients will have a naturally suppressed pituitary and thyroid anyway *before* you started them on thyroid (uhhh, that's why you decided to give them thyroid – remember?) – it's called aging. After you start them on thyroid supplementation you can check their free T4 but keep in mind if you check a TSH level it will probably be suppressed or low anyway. And that's all right because it will never come back unless you transplant them a new pituitary!

23. CoEnzyme Q10 is the last coenzyme in the energy pathway in the mitochondria of the cell and is inherently involved in the thyroid-energy pathways. If your patients are female or taking a little extra thyroid makes absolutely sure you give them adequate amounts of a high quality CoEnzyme Q10 supplement[132] (200 mgm a day at least).

24. Taking adequate amounts of T4/T3 thyroid supplementation will cause:
    A. Weight loss (WARNING: it is VERY illegal to prescribe for this purpose)
    B. Lowered cholesterol and lipids[133]
    C. Increased energy
    D. Warmer body temperature
    E. Increased immune resistance
    F. Increased cardiac output (decreased CHF)[134]
    G. Increased hair and nail thickness
    H. Improved cardiac output[135].
    I. No increased bone density loss (does not cause increased osteoporosis)[136].
    J. Improved fertility (females)[137].
    K. Clarity of thought and cognition improvements[138].
    L. T4 is almost exclusively the hormone that passes the blood brain barrier[139].

25. Some rare patients (usually women) have peripheral receptor sites (TR) that are not functioning nor binding hormone properly so they will cheat and take massive doses of thyroid hormone (9 to 15 grains a day!!!!). This will suppress the TSH level GREATLY so do not bother to get a TSH level on these patients. You will know who these are by the fact that they are very hyperactive and have lost a lot of weight. Make sure if you suspect someone's doing this that when you tell them to reduce their thyroid you also tell them to take a LOT (200 – 400 mgm a day) of high quality CoEnzymeQ10 (CoQ10)[140].

26. ZINC sometimes helps! The peripheral T3 receptor is thought to require zinc to adopt its biologically active conformation. Some of the effects of zinc deficiency, therefore, are due to loss of zinc from the T3 receptor and impairment of T3 action[141].

27. With excess exogenous or endogenous thyroid cardiac contractility and cardiac output are enhanced and systemic vascular resistance is decreased[142], while in hypothyroidism the opposite is true (you get increased vascular resistance, left ventricular hypertrophy)[143]. Which is better?

28. If you have a female patient who is incapable of getting pregnant or maintaining a pregnancy (and she's trying) and has tried everything check her thyroid – if in doubt, give her a mild dose (1/2 grain BID)[144].

29. Patients who take a combination of T4 and T3 (not just synthetic T4) have improved depression symptoms[145], feelings of well being, cardiac output, and quality of life – the goals of all worthwhile clinicians[146].

30. The psychiatric community has used T3 (Cytomel® - liothyronine) for years for mood stabilization and depression and mania with great effect and they rarely look at any lab work[147] and often usually use supraphysiologic doses.

31. If you have a patient with PCOS put them on thyroid supplementation and watch the great improvement[148].

32. You need to reassess all those chronic fatigue patients with odd annoying complaints that you historically have just hated seeing in your office – check their TSH, Free T3, and Free T4 with a

high level of suspicion. If in doubt act like a psychiatrist and put them on a little thyroid hormone (dessicated) anyway[149].

33. Too fatigued to exercise? Think of subclinical hypothyroidism[150].

34. Young and suffering from specific memory loss issues and feeling just generally lousy and seen numerous physicians without good effect? Try them on a low dose of dessicated thyroid[151]. And there is usually NO adverse effect to higher dose treatment[152]!!

35. Most cases of fibromyalgia fall into the category of type II (hormone resistant) hypothyroidism. Preliminary evidence suggests that serum hyaluronic acid is a simple, inexpensive, sensitive, and specific test that identifies fibromyalgia. The thyroid-resistant disorders might be treatable with *experimentally proven treatment of supraphysiologic doses of thyroid hormone*. Someone with total thyroid failure may have mild symptoms compared to someone who has moderate thyroid failure[153].

36. Know that the element selenium (200 mcg a day at most) assists the deiodinase enzyme in converting T4 to T3 (use if T4 is good but T3 is low).

37. Recently hypothyroidism has been associated as a risk factor for Colorectal and Breast cancers!

38. Even most of the experts think you should treat subclinical (read overt symptom free) hypothyroidism[154].

39. Overt symptoms of subclinical hypothyroidism include hypercholesterolemia, coronary disease, cerebrovascular disease, plus neuropsychiatric manifestations of mood depression, memory and cognition impairment and declining sense of well being, and improves with both T4 and T3[155]. Why, as caregivers, would we not treat this?

40. Though endocrinologists claim it, TSH should not be used to evaluate the severity of thyroid failure. It's the free T3 hormone that affects the peripheral tissues at the cellular level[156] NOT the circulating TSH.

41. Rarely you will get a patient who's incredibly sensitive to any thyroid hormone[157] (despite lab and patient appearing as if hypothyroid) and they go into tachycardia or severe anxiety with the smallest doses. Just beware.

42. Remember -- treat the patient not the lab (unless level's are not optimized then give them a little extra)[158]. ☺

Checking Levels

This might be a paradigm shift for you in thyroid care and thought. Good!

Forget everything you know about thyroid problems and start over. Know that TSH levels have zero impact on the way a patient feels.

Critical Point #1: Treat the patient's clinical symptoms not their lab. Remember that we're "clinicians" not "labicians." The lab levels serve only as a guide post but you have to use your brain to interpret them correctly.

Critical Point #2: Your patient's symptoms stem from the level of Free T3[159] (or lack thereof) in their system – not from their level of TSH or T4[160].

Critical Point #3: Look first and mainly at your patient's Free T3 levels[161].

Critical Point #4: A low but normal level of Free T3 is clinically significantly low, especially because most patients will also have concurrent symptoms of fatigue and lethargy. From another perspective that Free T3 level is really lower than it appears because most of these patients have additional T3 receptor failure on their peripheral tissues[162].

Critical Point #5: If your patient's Free T3 levels are normal and they still have symptoms of hypothyroidism think thyroid T3 receptor failure on peripheral cells. This is a common finding in the elderly and people with chronic illnesses[163] such as chronic renal failure (CKD) and they can have low T3 and T4 levels with normal thyroid-stimulating hormone (TSH) levels[164].

Critical Point #6: Don't be afraid to optimize their level of Free T3 to 3.9-4.0 pg/ml or above. If they have receptor failure they may need this extra exogenous T3 and T4[165] to feel well[166].

Critical Point #7: A small percentage of hypothyroid patients will have thyroid sensitivity in their hypothyroidism making their cardiac tissue exquisitely sensitive to any level of thyroid causing atrial fibrillation[167], SVTs, angina, and other cardiac abnormalities. Start these patients on a tiny does (1/4 grain of dessicated thyroid) twice a day to begin with.

Critical Point #8: Remember if they have also any thyroid 2'deiodinase[168] (D2) failure or malfunction (not uncommon in the elderly) they will not convert a significant amount of exogenous or endogenous T4 to the active hormone (T3)[169], no matter how much synthetic T4 (levo-thyroxine) you or their endocrinologist gives them, thus their T3 levels will remain low or low normal, while their Free T4 will remain very high and their TSH may be suppressed or elevated. Remember – look at the Free T3 level first and mainly!

Critical Point #9: MALPRACTICE WARNING! If all their levels are very low (Free T3, Free T4 and TSH) and they're acting goofy or psychotic BE VERY CAREFUL – these patients have an emergent mixedematous coma and need to be admitted to the hospital. You will treat these patients with kid gloves very slowly and carefully because they are extremely sensitive to thyroid hormone (starting them on ¼ grain a day of dessicated thyroid and only increasing it every 4 or 5 days).

In general, check a TSH, Free Serum T4, and Free Serum T3 (always focusing on the Free T3 level) to begin with when you first evaluate the patient. Remember that a relatively low or normal free T4 and free T3 with a low TSH can indicate a thyroid inadequacy.

After optimizing therapies you can check their Free T3 but keep in mind if you check a TSH level it will probably be suppressed (this is alright because you've optimized their thyroid levels).

Thyroid Practice Gems

A. Ideally order it from your compounding pharmacy by saying on the script:

Compounded T3/T4 Capsule (Armour® formula)

B. Start low (1/2 to 1 grain per day) of the dessicated natural form of thyroid (an encapsulated forms works best).

C. 1 Grain = 60 mgm

D. Do not try to use a sustained release thyroid or you will get unusually low levels despite treatment with ever larger doses.

E. Average daily dose is about 2 grains in males and 3 grains in females.

F. If they have RTH (Resistance to Thyroid Hormone due to faulty receptors) don't be fooled by a low TSH. As a matter of fact it is pointless (and confusing) to continue to check TSH levels in these patients. Just give them more dessicated thyroid.

G. Never ever give thyroid for weight loss (even though weight normalization tends to occur when the dose is appropriate) – this is illegal.

H. NOTE: MALPRACTICE WARNING! Always watch for angina or CAD or SVT arrhythmia problems in these patients. Could be from too much thyroid or paradoxically even too little thyroid.

If you give thyroid then always give CoEnzyme Q10 along with it, especially in patients who have CHF and *especially* in patients taking a statin.

Usually you can ignore the lab values on the lab form – go with the optimized values which we've listed.

Iodine Capsules

For Iodine Deficiency Disorder and the subsequent goiter, give iodine capsules to alleviate[170]. This situation can also cause either subclinical or overt hypothyroidism so test accordingly.

Possible Side Effects of Too Much Thyroid (Exogenous Hyperthyroidism)

Hypocholesterolemia[171]

Right Ventricular Hypertrophy, atrial fibrillation (4.00%), ventricular premature beats (2.77%), paroxysmal supraventricular tachycardia (2.23%), atrial flutter (1.00%).

Congestive heart failure occurred in 10.42% of the cases in one review[172].

Dementia (long-term extreme hyperthyroidism according to the Rotterdam Study)[173]

Refractory SVT[174] (supraventricular tachycardia)

F./G. Estrogen/Progesterone HRT

With the reporting of HERS[175] and WHI[176] studies, hormone replacement therapy (HRT) has been saddled with several erroneous beliefs that we will quickly explode and then it is our hope that you will consider the much more physiological and natural approach of replacement therapy with modern biologically identical human hormones.

HRT Erroneous Belief #1

"Estrogen and progesterone were the hormones used in those studies and they're bad for me, right doctor, they cause cancer, heart attacks, and strokes, right?"

Wrong AND right.

Estrogen and progesterone as created in the human body – natural estrogens and progesterones – were not used in either of those studies. Synthetic progestational agents that are foreign to your body and very inflammatory[177] for your blood vessels and heart were used in both studies as were conjugated equine estrogen -- taken from pregnant mare's urine – another problematic hormone substance for human females. Both of these have been proven to be injurious when given long term before these studies so smarter physicians in general are not sure why they were used in these important studies. Conjugated equine estrogen (Premarin®), used in both studies, contains some estradiol and some estriol (which partially converts to estrone in the human body) but seems to contain other hormones that are not conducive to long term women's health – there lies the problems.

HRT Erroneous Belief #2

"So, doctor, if you won't give me those hormones because they're so bad (not that I would let you any way) then what do you suggest?"

Good question. For more than a decade there have been widely available in this country biologically identical human hormones that give you excellent benefits without minimal effects when given properly and who's levels can be tracked with blood tests (which cannot be done with synthetic progestational agents) and adjusted accordingly. These hormones are identical to what every patient makes in their bodies.

HRT Erroneous Belief #3

"But doesn't estrogen cause breast cancer?"

The conjugated equine estrogens in Premarin® contain carcinogenic equilin and equilenin which can cause breast cancer (the 17 alpha-dihydroderivatives of equilenin and equilin -- 15% of the CEE components -- have a non-estrogenic or even an anti-estrogenic effect on breast tissue)[178].

On the other hand, biologically identical human estrogens have not been associated in any studies with breast cancer but regardless, they should always be properly opposed with human progesterone.

HRT Erroneous Belief #4

"So taking Premarin® won't give me any human estrogens? Wouldn't a natural estrogen be better? "

Not true. Patients who take the so-called natural estrogens (soy and plant based) rarely if ever reach optimized protective levels of estradiol[179] (>50 pg/mL[180]), while patients who take Premarin® almost always have levels beyond these therapeutic levels when randomly checked. The trouble with conjugated equine estrones is what they carry with them – equilin and equilenin and their derivatives which are associated with breast cancer and exaggerated potency in the hepatic system[181]. But if a choice had to be made, Premarin® is far superior to "natural" plant based estrogens because of concentration and estrogen load.

F. Estrogen (Usually Estradiol and Estriol)

(Note: Only for surgical or FSH-elevated (>50 mIU/ml[182]) confirmed menopause.)

Human estrogen is produced in four different forms[183] – estrone (E1), estradiol (E2), estriol (E3), and estetrol (E4 -- in pregnancy only). Estradiol is the most physiologically and biologically active and the one which offers the most protection and benefits —it also converts to estrone which, along with estradiol, also converts to estriol, so technically and theoretically (if the patient is young enough to have all their CYP3A7 cytochrome P-450 16-hydroxylation liver conversion enzymes remaining intact[184]) it can be the only estrogen you need to give. But usually this form of HRT is given orally or transdermally (only in certain situations) as a bi-estrogen, or BiEst, containing both estradiol and estriol (many people believe that estriol protects against cancer but there have been no studies to prove this) or more specifically human 17-β-estradiol which can also be given in a compounded form or as Estrace ® at 1 mgm a day which usually gives high enough levels to give proper cardiovascular protection[185].

Dosing and Manner

Most often it should be given orally in a capsule (safer for the heart and breasts but slightly higher risk of gallstones[186]) as compounded Bi-Est in the morning consisting of a beginning dose of 0.5 mgm of estriol and 1.0 mgm of estradiol. We also know now that you can give your patients pure compounded 17-β-estradiol (E2) at either 1.0-2.0 mgm or as Estrace® 1.0 mgm a day. The estradiol level can be raised to 1.5

mgm, or 2.0 mgm or decreased to 0.5 mgm but always keep it (you can choose not to give the estriol for a number of good reasons).

Note that estriol (E3) is the breakdown product of estradiol (E2) and because of this does not actually have to be given.

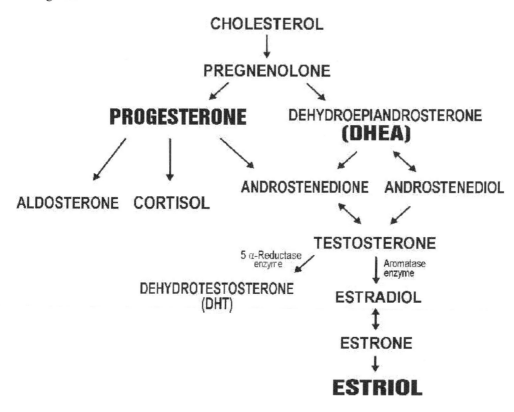

Oral Estrogen CVD Warnings

ORAL ESTROGEN WARNING #1 -- Prothrombin 20210G→A Variant Warning

Do not EVER give oral estradiol to women who are *postmenopausal with essential hypertension* because a high **percentage of these particular hypertensive women will have a prothrombin clotting factor genetic variant**[187] (mutation) and could suffer from VTE/DVT, MI (332 % increased risk[188]), or stroke[189]. Though oral is clearly the best option, with these particular patients instead, give them a transdermal estradiol patch[190] (to protect their skin and mucosa and some bone protection only but at least transdermal will protect that[191]).

(For the technically minded this is the Prothrombin 20210G→A Variant[192].)

Do not give or allow to be given oral estrogen to these women (if these are your patients stop the oral estrogen and switch them to transdermal BiEst or the Climara® patch).

ORAL ESTROGEN WARNING #2 – The Oral Estradiol Window!

We do know from HERS, the Nurses' Health Study, and the WHI that there is a **window of opportunity for safely starting oral estradiol**[193] in postmenopausal women starting within a year after they become menopausal (average age in USA is 51) and going up to age 60 after which they are at increased risk for the first year of oral estradiol for a myocardial infarction[194]. Use extreme caution and have them sign an informed consent/release if they still want oral estradiol and are willing to face the risks involved. Otherwise use transdermal Bi-Est or transdermal Estrace® or an estradiol ring in these women (see below).

We know however those endogenous AND exogenous estrogens, such as estradiol, protect the cardiovascular system, and several observational studies and a few small clinical studies conducted *in healthy and younger postmenopausal women* (i.e. under 60) support this hypothesis[195].

However if these older women are already more than a year on oral estrogens or have a long history of being on estrogen it is far more beneficial and cardioprotective, neuroprotective, and osteoprotective for them to continue the oral estrogens at this point.

Article In Support of Oral Estrogen Warnings

Read the following landmark articles if you disagree with these warnings.

Differential association of oral and transdermal oestrogen-replacement therapy with venous thrombonembolism risk by Pierre-Yves Scarabin, et al in The Lancet 2003; 362:428-432.

Hormone Replacement Therapy, Prothrombotic Mutations, and the Risk of Incident Nonfatal Myocardial Infarction in Postmenopausal Women by Bruce M. Psaty, MD, PhD et al. in JAMA. 2001;285:906-913.

Alternatives to Oral Estrogen Therapy by Valerie L. Baker, MD in Obstetrics and Gynecology Clinics of North America, Vol. 21, No. 2, June 1994, pp. 271-97.

Levels

For a NEWLY menopausal woman you want treated estradiol levels to be 75-100 pg/mL or slightly greater.

For an OLDER menopausal woman you want treated estradiol levels to be >50 pg/mL or slightly greater (JT Hargrove et al suggested levels of 50-150 pg/ml[196] but we'd keep it below 100 pg/ml to prevent estrogen predominance symptoms).

Levels should be maintained above 50 pg/ml (to 100 pg/ml) to keep patients feeling the best physically[197] and psychologically[198].

In humans, the epidemiological studies have shown that premenopausal women have a much lower mortality from atherosclerotic cardiovascular disease than men, suggesting that sex hormones might have a cardioprotective effect[199].

Simple Point on Biologically Identical Human Estrogens

Bio-identical Human Estrogens
(not patentable because we all manufacture in our body)

----------**vs.**---------------

Synthetic Estrogens (patentable)

Any questions?

Effects of No Estrogen

1. Vaginal dryness and atrophy[200]
2. Urinary incontinence[201]
3. Hot flashes[202] that do not resolve with progesterone use supraphysiological doses
4. Temperature dysregulation
5. Balance problems
6. Sagging wrinkled skin[203]
7. Sagging breasts[204]
8. Epidermal thinning, declining dermal collagen content, diminished skin moisture, decreased laxity, and impaired wound healing[205]
9. Fatigue[206]
10. Depression[207]
11. Mood swings[208]
12. Declining libido to no libido
13. Acceleration of glomerulosclerosis
14. Osteoporosis[209]
15. Coronary artery disease[210]
16. Sexual dysfunction[211]
17. Tooth loss and receding gums (always attractive)[212].
18. Alzheimer's Disease[213]

Benefits Of Human Bi-Estrogen (ERT: Estradiol and Estriol: E2 and E3) or Estradiol (E2 or Estrace®)

Estrogen supplementation prevents macular degeneration[214].

Estrogen supplementation prevents cataracts[215].

Estrogen supplementation prevents memory loss and Alzheimer's disease[216].

Estrogen prevents osteoporosis[217].

Estrogen prevents against vaginal atrophy, dry eyes, and skin wrinkling and increases skin thickness in the process[218].

Estradiol is cardioprotective by decreasing LDL levels and elevating HDL levels[219] [220].

Estradiol protects against Ischemic Stroke (contrary to the WHI[221]) (by preventing activation of neutrophils by TNF alpha, thus decreasing the expression of adhesion molecules, the adhesion of neutrophils - endothelial cells, and hence the risk of ischemic stroke)[222].

Evidence clearly establishes that estradiol is a potent neuroprotective and neurotrophic factor in the adult: it influences memory and cognition, decreases the risk and delays the onset of neurological diseases such as Alzheimer's disease, and attenuates the extent of cell death that results from brain injuries such as cerebrovascular stroke and neurotrauma[223].

Direct Antiatherosclerotic Effects[224]
Inhibits deposition of LDL and its byproducts in blood vessel walls
Decreases lipoprotein-induced arterial smooth muscle proliferation
Decreases foam cell formation in vessel wall
Reduces arterial cholesterol ester influx and hydrolysis
Decreases elastin and collagen production and accumulation
Inhibits platelet aggregation
Increases prostacyclin production by endothelium and arterial smooth muscle cells
Decreases thromboxane A2 formation
Reduces oxidation of LDL

Protects against vascular injury
Accelerates endothelial cell growth and inhibits apoptosis
Inhibits proliferation of smooth muscle cells
Estrogen-related genes ameliorate negative effects of collagen, E-selectin, vascular endothelial growth factor, and fibrinogen proteins

Direct Vasodilatory Effects[225]

Decreases vascular tone
Modulates release of vasoconstrictors and vasodilators by vascular endothelium, thereby decreasing vascular reactivity
Modulates ionic channels in smooth muscle cell membranes of vessels and cardiac cells
Modulates release of vasoactive substances and neurotransmitters
Modulates vasoactive neurotransmitter release at presynaptic junctions
Increases vasodilating and antiplatelet aggregation factors in endothelium
Increases vasodilation by nonendothelium-dependent factor
Estrogen-related genes ameliorate negative effects of endothelin, prostacyclin synthase, and endothelial nitric oxide

Systemic Effects[226]

Decreases total cholesterol and LDL levels; increases HDL levels
Increases inotropic actions of the heart
Improves glucose metabolism; decreases circulating insulin levels
Lowers blood pressure through vasodilatation
Reduces plasminogen-activator inhibitor
Decreases fibrinogen

Side Effects of Estrogen Dominance or Unopposed Estrogen

1. In PeriMenopausal patients* with estrogen dominance[227]:
    A. Premenopausal mood swings, depression
    B. Breast swelling, fibrocystic disease
    C. Craving sweets
    D. Heavy or irregular menses
    E. Sleep disturbances: Insomnia or fatigue
    F. Uterine fibroids
    G. Weight gain, fat deposition on hips and thighs
    H. Acne and skin breaks out
    I. Water retention, edema

*This can go on for years starting in a patient's late 30's to until menopause in their early 50s – so realize that the estrogen dominance effect can be overwhelming and very long lasting (overwhelming their risk factors for breast and endometrial cancer) – so offset with adequate human progesterone, please!

2. **The Five B's of Estrogen Dominance** (can occur with PMS* [Pre-Menstrual Syndrome] or with PMS* [PeriMenopausal Symptoms]):
    A. **Backache**
    B. **Bleeding** (excessively)
    C. **Bloating**
    D. **Breast** (tenderness)
    E. **Bitchiness**
    (Okay, at the behest of well known gynecologists let's add a tentative 6ᵗʰ B – Uterine FiBroids)

*Treat both PMSs the same way – this is from estrogen dominance or over-production (which can also predispose them to breast cancer and endometrial *hyperplasia [ask if their mom had this and* *did she have breast CA or uterine cancer]*) – give them 100 mgm progesterone triturates for sublingual dissolution for whenever they start to have these symptoms. Help them! And if 1 doesn't work try 2 each day! And if 2 doesn't work try 3! And if 3 doesn't work try 4! (Remember, *oral* human progesterone or P4 is a sedative and soporific while this is not true of the sublingual triturates.)

3. Breast Cancer[228]
4. Endometrial Cancer[229]
5. Thrombosis[230]
6. Weight gain[231] – debatable (exercise helps – do lots of it!)
7. Fluid retention[232] – use Dyazide
8. Uterine Fibroids (Uterine Leiomyomas)[233]
9. Migraine Headache[234]
10. Gallstones – when given orally[235]
11. Heart Attack (HERS study[236] – wrong kinds of estrogen though [i.e. CEE])
12. Tooth loss and jaw resorption[237]
13. Depressed mood[238]

How to fix?

If premenopausal or perimenopausal or even premenstrual syndrome (all the kinds of PMS out there) give – give them 100 mgm progesterone triturates (see Progesterone info below) for sublingual dissolution for whenever they start to have these symptoms. Help them!

If you get these symptoms in some one who's post-menopausal and on modern HRT, lower the dose of estradiol in the BiEst you are giving. If that doesn't work keep dose low but cut out the Estriol (E3) portion.

Practice Gems on Estrogen Supplementation

1. Protect your patient from cancers, cataracts and heart disease – it is your obligation – give them proper HRT protection.

2. Take E2 and E3 as a micronized capsule. Give them Estrace® 1 mg a day if their insurance will cover it. Give them generic Estrace® if they are financially struggling and have no insurance.

3. Ask your patients if they want to be dried up like a prune and have incredibly wrinkled skin, no teeth, and no sex – or would they like some estrogen?

4. **Pre-/Perimenopausal Situations**: look at FSH levels which porpoise (go up and down). If premenopausal you can give progesterone only (1 tablet a day) – they make plenty of estrogen naturally. No use taking or checking levels of estradiol or progesterone in these patients. If perimenopausal, check FSH levels and if high then treat, if not high (if low) you can use progesterone – no harm in giving progesterone to an anovulatory perimenopausal woman. If they want to bleed (ask them) just stop the progesterone – if they don't want to bleed continue the progesterone. After 3 to 6 months stop the progesterone, after one month check a FSH level to see where they are.

5. Does you no good to measure pre-menopausal estradiol and progesterone levels because you don't know where they are in their cycle. Check FSH and LH levels instead if you are so concerned.

6. You can diagnose menopause by symptoms – if no menses for six (6) months it's menopause. This goes for almost any age, any symptoms. If they request it you better suspect it. Measure the FSH and LH (menopause if both are >50).

7. Use human biologically identical hormones not equine urine estrones which (as we've said repeatedly) contain 17 androgenic and carcinogenic agents.

8. Tri-estrogen combination was tried first but too many side effects (our female patients make enough estrone anyway) so use a BiEst (bi-estrogen or two estrogens) containing both estradiol (20%) and estriol (80%) in doses such as 1.5 mgm, 2.0 mgm, or 2.5 mgm (usually contains only 0.5 mgm estriol). Even easier, just use estradiol (such as Estrace® 1 mg).

9. Do not use estrone. Not breast tissue friendly. This is also already created in the stomach lining to such an extent that most women are never short of estrone.

10. If you have a patient on HRT aggressively communicate the need for PAP and breast mammograms – every 2 years according to the American Cancer Association and ACOG (if they are past age 40) but annually if in your modern HRT. Send out letters. Do everything. Send out 13 letters if necessary!

    MALPRACTICE WARNING: Do not refill HRT unless they comply!

11. Don't guess. Check levels! **Optimal estradiol level is 50-100 pg/ml.** You can get annoying side effects if above 100 (breast tenderness, vaginal bleeding, bloating, breaking out), but must be at least 50 pg/ml to give protection.

12. No need to cycle estradiol after menopause – give every day!

13. If they have had their uterus, ovaries removed then give them everything – BiEst, Testosterone, DHEA, Progesterone. Save their lives!

14. MALPRACTICE WARNING: Absolute contraindications – history of clots, thrombosis, emboli, or HTN (hypertension). DO NOT GIVE THESE PATIENTS ORAL ESTROGEN! Give them an estradiol patch (Climara®) (and Niaspan® 500 mgm BID) or an estrogen ring (see below). (Note: patch does not help as strongly against CV disease[239] as oral.)

15. If they have hot flashes that are not resolved go to BID with the BiEst or Estrace® for 6 months or so until the symptoms resolve.

16. If they do not have hot flashes until after you start the BiEst (or estradiol) then double the dose for 6 months or so, but if this does not resolve the hot flashes then switch them to a topical patch such as Climara® or Yasmin® (the least androgenic BCPs on the market and for that reason, as this book is written, a Dr. Purser favorite) as BCP can also decrease hot flashes, so try if you're desperate. Know, though, that hot flashes are actually usually caused by perimenopausal decline of the hormone *inhibin*[240].

    The other opinion in regards to hot flashes being that in some women catecholestrogens (estrogen metabolites) from oral estrogen[241] "resetting the thermostat" is to blame for the hot flashes[242] – if you suspect this is the case switch them to the Climara® patch for great 24 hour coverage – it's worth a try.

17. Be aware that (very rarely) they can start ovulating on the natural hormones and can get pregnant – warn them if they are younger postmenopausal patients!!!

18. If the patient is past the window for HRT (age 50-60 years) or has hypertension (thus a prothrombotic risk) use a vaginal estradiol ring or tablet. Femring® and Vagifem® tablets give proper estradiol levels similar to the Climara® patch while Estring® is for those women with breast cancer, DVT, or MI histories who are having localized vaginal

issues (urinary frequency, dry vagina, incontinence, etc) and in who you do not want circulating estrogens. The Femring®/Vagifem® option can treat hot flashes in some patients (in the occasional instances when progesterone does not).

19. Warning! Estriol (E3) tends to cause bloating or the feeling of bloating and if this occurs among your HRT patients stop their estriol first. Give a diuretic next (i.e. Dyazide®).

20. There is absolutely no need to check estradiol levels in men. What is being said on the internet is WRONG! If true, at what level would they like the estradiol level to rise before intervention with anastrozole is begun? *[This is a Socratic question.]* There is no answer to this because Estradiol is cardioprotective and prevents against strokes in men[243] . Leave it alone unless they get significant breast enlargement!

Vaginal Atrophy (One More Time)

Vaginal atrophy is far easier to prevent than to treat but if you wish to treat it effectively make sure your patient's level of testosterone is adequate as this seems to be the best way to promote vaginal moisture[244] and even can cause a slight discharge (please tell your patients to wear a pad if this becomes annoying as too much moisture is far superior and healthier than having the Sahara Desert down there). This urogenital atrophy can also lead to a decline in sexual desire and functionality so give them testosterone[245].

Second if the oral estrogen is not working then add a local estrogen[246] (according to their histories and needs) such as:

PREFERRED (if you are also giving oral E2) →Estring® → ONLY localized levels of estrogen so gives vaginal protection only!

Femring® → Circulating levels of estrogen so vaginal/osteoporosis protection

Vagifem® tablets → Circulating levels of estrogen so vaginal/osteoporosis protection

NOTE: these avoid the FIRST PASS EFFECT in the liver and so do not effect lipids or give cardioprotection as well as oral estradiol. If they are at risk for heart disease give them the oral estradiol if it's safe (i.e. if they are not past the window[247] and no hypertension [Prothrombin variant[248]])!

Preventing Vaginal Atrophy Prevents Stress Incontinence, Too!

Note that this vaginal or urogenital atrophy can lead to stress incontinence which is, as we've said, a LOT easier to prevent than to treat, once it occurs. If this is starting to occur in one of your patients (or all of your patients) push the estradiol levels a little higher OR add the local estradiol rings or tablets to prevent this problem. Save these women years of misery!

Osteoporosis Prevention

How important is this?

Very. The increasing epidemic of osteoporosis-related fractures constitutes a major public health problem in the United States. With a few preventive measures such as identification of risk factors, careful examination, and a few simple diagnostic tests, prevention of osteoporosis during the teen and early adult years is far superior to any treatment for older individuals[249].

Fractures from osteoporosis are a *major* killer of elderly women and it's our fault if we let one of our patients get so osteoporotic that they fracture something and die. We are generally NOT doing a very good job of this[250].

It's our fault if they need Fosamax®, too. If this occurs we have not handled these patients appropriately.

Sadly, 54 % of women have osteopenia, 30 % have osteoporosis. 97% of free living women >71 years of age and 99% of nursing home women have a Vitamin D deficiency[251].

Diagnosis of Osteoporosis: Get baseline dual-energy x-ray absorptiometry[252] (DeXA which is the gold standard for measuring bone density) to diagnose. Repeat the BMD (DeXA) every two years (that's how fast it changes and how often Medicare will pay for it).

Get a NTX (2nd urine of the morning) to track more effectively (changes within a few months)[253]. Can get this annually. NTX tells you if there's immediate ongoing loss or gain of bone mineral density (BMD). Read the literature.

Check estradiol[254] and progesterone levels, too.

You can also get the main circulating Vitamin D levels (25 OHD or 25–Hydroxy-Vitamin D)[255]. Calcium levels are not helpful, while knowing their average daily calcium dose is (should be 1500 mg premenopause and 1000 mg per day postmenopause.

Treatment of Osteoporosis:

Vitamin D3 (cholecalciferol) is more potent than D2 (ergocalciferol): Improves osteoporosis[256]. Decreases fall risk (this and other benefits are covered later in this chapter).

Vitamin K2 is more potent than K1: Promotes the synthesis of proteins involved with calcium utilization, increases absorption of calcium from the gut, decreases fracture risk.[257]

Both Sexes > 65 yrs of age:

*Use Alendronate (Fosamax®) EVERY time[258] just to protect you from lawsuits etc. Although biphosphonates have been shown to reduce bone resorption and inhibit osteoclasts, their effectiveness seems to be best for treatment in women with osteoporosis and they do not appear to work as well as estrogens in prevention of osteoporosis[259]. Although Quandt and colleagues[260] have found that alendronate therapy in women with osteopenia reduces vertebral fracture risk, Schousboe and colleagues performed a cost-effectiveness analysis to estimate the cost per quality-adjusted life-year (QALY) gained from a five-year alendronate (Fosamax) regimen in women 55 to 75 years of age with osteopenia and no additional risk factors, the final result suggesting that it costs more than a reasonable amount[261].

Let us restate that – alendronate is *not* cost effective to use.

Ibandronate (Boniva®) is a biphosphonate that can be taken daily or monthly. The daily dosage has been shown to decrease vertebral fractures in women with osteoporosis and a history of previous vertebral fractures. It has *not* been shown to reduce the risk of hip fracture or other nonvertebral fracture, nor to reduce fractures in women without prior fracture. *Ibandronate has not been compared directly with other biphosphonates or with adequate daily doses of calcium and vitamin D[262].*

Let us restate that – alendronate and ibandronate just reduce the incidence of fractures and reduce the bone loss BUT they do not increase the BMD – they just slow the rate of loss and are not cost effective (unlike HRT and Vitamin D/Cal Mag Aspartate).

As a matter of fact, no biphosphonate has been compared with adequate doses of calcium and vitamin D[263] [264] which we know are inexpensive, side effect free (actually taking adequate doses of either gives you a huge list of benefits), and very effective[265] in combination.

Biphosphonates have been shown to slow the demineralization of patient's bones but studies have not clearly shown that biphosphonates reverse bone loss unlike hormones[266]! Read the studies! HRT is more much cheaper and more effective than alendronate according to the experts! Do your job, physicians!

But to prevent easy malpractice suits, put every osteoporotic patient you have on Fosamax® because even the attorneys won't understand what we just said. Understand?

*Oral Estradiol with appropriate optimized serum levels prevents and improves and *even reverses* osteopenia and osteoporosis[267]. Also, improves muscle strength and decreases fall risk[268] (again important). Same with Vitamin D!

*Take Calcium(334 mg) with Magnesium(166 mg) in a Cal-Mag Aspartate combination at 2–5 pills per day[269] to reduce osteopenia/-porosis. This combination also reduces hsCRP!

*Vitamin D3 (800-1000 IU/day) with Vitamin K1 [or Phytonadione] (100 mcg/day) or K2 [Menaquinone] 45-90 mcg/day[270]. *[More simply have your patients take 1000 - 2000 U Vitamin D3 a day and 1 mg Vitamin K – have this compounded for your patients. Review the Vitamin D section towards the end of this chapter.]*

*All calcium carbonate contains high lead levels so use a Calcium Citrate or Cal-Mag Aspartate supplement[271].

*For optimal Zinc and Magnesium and safety take a better vitamin but one with no iron[272] and no copper[273] (very hard to find) – these act as very detrimental pro-oxidants especially in people over 40. So avoid them by using the Vitaline Green Formula®.

*Increased fruits and vegetables (i.e. as in the DASH diet) reduce osteoporosis[274].

*Take B12/Folate to reduce homocysteine levels -- lower homocysteine levels reduce fracture risk, too[275].

G. Progesterone (P4)

Progesterone (4-pregnene-3, 20-dione or P4 in this case[276]) is the "feel good" hormone of pregnancy. We are strictly talking about naturally occurring biologically identical human progesterone – not synthetic progestational agents such as progestin, medroxyprogesterone acetate, or norethisterone – these are not the natural progesterone and are very problematic and side effect intensive (they have almost exactly the opposite side effects when compared to the benefits of natural progesterone).

Known Side Effects From Taking Medroxyprogesterone (Provera® or MPA)
(Studies are legion, look at Pub Med for more supporting articles)
MPA is a teratogen and cannot be used in pregnancy[277].
MPA increases cholesterol and increases risk of heart disease[278].
MPA increases foam cell formation, endothelial inflammation, plaque formation, strokes and heart attacks[279]
.
MPA is carcinogenic and causes breast cancer[280] (see PEPI[281] trial).
MPA has no effect on osteoporosis (i.e. does not help)[282].
MPA is associated with side effects of increased bleeding, bloating, and depression[283].
MPA provides a serum progesterone level of zero – it is immeasurable as progesterone.

Why? MPA IS NOT PROGESTERONE[284]!

Dosing of P4 and Vehicle

Usual dose of micronized P4 is 100 mgm a day in a triturate or flavored troche. To avoid first pass effect in the liver[285] you dissolve either in your mouth under your tongue (SUBLINGUALLY) until completely dissolved, avoiding drinking or eating anything ten minutes before or after.

Levels

This may be a new concept for you but, yes, you can and should get serum progesterone levels -- monthly until they are at a therapeutic level (> 10 ng/ml – 20 ng/ml) then at least annually thereafter.

"Normal" P4 Values[286]

- Female (pre-ovulation): less than 1 ng/mL
- Female (mid-cycle): 5 to 20 ng/mL
- Male: less than 1 ng/mL
- Postmenopausal: less than 1 ng/mL
- 1st trimester: 11.2-90.0 ng/mL
- 2nd trimester: 25.6-89.4 ng/mL
- 3rd trimester: 48.4-42.5 ng/mL

Initial Levels

On initial exam most patients will have zero progesterone levels if they are menopausal. They may be taking some OTC natural progesterone product which might give them a little in their serum (but this would require a LOT of natural OTC progesterone). *[They could bathe in a natural progesterone cream 24 hours a day and not get therapeutic levels.]*

Ideal Levels

You want progesterone levels to be 10 ng/mL or greater (up to but not above 20 ng/ml) for optimal protection from breast[287] and uterine cancer. We disagree with Hargrove in not regularly checking levels as our experience has shown that if levels are too high for a long time you can get significant weight gain and maximal acinar and minimal ductal and stromal cell proliferation of the breast and vagina[288].

Problem Levels

There are no levels that are too high because in pregnancy you can see levels that are in the 200-400 ng/ml range. But for the above reasons keep them below 20 ng/ml.

If levels climb above 50 or 100 ng/ml? **Look for pregnancy!**

Benefits of Biologically Identical Human Progesterone (P4)

P4, when levels are optimized, aggressively and effectively:

1. Lowers cholesterol *[at 200 mgm of micronized progesterone a day in one PEPI study arm[289] – sound familiar?]*(Especially when given in conjunction with E2)[290].
2. Elevates HDL levels (hard to do)[291].
3. Decreases foam cell formation[292], endothelial inflammation, plaque formation, and thus strokes and heart attacks[293].
4. Decreases breast density and thus breast cancer[294].
5. Increases bone density preventing osteoporosis and related fractures[295].
6. Prevents and treats endometrial hyperplasia (use triple or quadruple the usual dose)[296].
7. If you give enough, progesterone almost always halts uterine bleeding (cyclical bleeding)[297].

8. Can act as a hypersomniac (sleep aid) if you give 100 mgm at night orally for sleep[298] problems. Orally administered progesterone may have advantages over other routes of administration in the treatment of premenstrual syndrome (PMS) because of substantially higher levels of the anxiolytic metabolites 5 alpha and 5 beta pregnanolone[299] which also cause drowsiness[300].
9. Oral P4 also treats peri-menopausal symptoms (also called PMS) in the same manner (give double or triple the usual dose for about a week)[301].
10. Remember -- an oral micronized progesterone given sublingually has improved bioavailability and much fewer reported side effects compared with synthetic progestins[302].
11. P4, when given with estradiol, improves the quality of life according to a Mayo Clinic report[303]
12. Improves libido (along with testosterone)[304].
13. Synthetic progestins, on the other hand, often cause androgenic side effects (acne, body and facial hair), depression, and weight gain. Micronized progesterone is devoid of the androgenic effects on the lipid profile seen with MPA and other synthetic progestational agents; for that reason, it may be preferable in HRT protocols for perimenopausal and postmenopausal women[305].
14. Men should not take progesterone unless they are a sex offender in jail[306] (see below).

Progesterone Practice Gems and Problem Solving

A. Whether capsule, troche, or triturate give 100 mgm of human progesterone (P4) every morning.

B. Normal premenopausal progesterone levels (in women) are 4-25 ng/ml. Optimal levels are a little tighter at 10-20 ng/ml.

C. Only get serum progesterone levels not salivary or urinary levels[307] (because they are completely inaccurate). This salivary approach, though highly touted on the internet, is not supported in the literature as being accurate.

D. Usually biologically identical human progesterone is given as a flavored triturate or troche under the tongue until it dissolves (no chewing or swallowing if they can help it and do not drink pr eat ten minutes before or after taking).

E. PROBLEM: One of your patients you've started on HRT comes in for her annual exam and on her Pap smear you get *endometrial hyperplasia* – what should you do? Get an intravaginal ultrasound[308] – looking for the endometrial stripe (or a polyp, adenoma, fibroid, cancer), if<5 mm then you're okay – keep treating with HRT with extra progesterone[309]. If >5 mm then stop HRT and refer to an Ob-Gyn.

F. BLEEDING PROBLEM: Your postmenopausal patient has been taking her natural BiEst and Human Progesterone exactly as you prescribed and suddenly she starts bleeding vaginally (a period??!?!) – what do you do? Stop BiEst and double her progesterone (P4) until bleeding stops then go back on BiEst but keep progesterone at double.

1. After three months you go back to standard doses of progesterone. Then she starts bleeding vaginally again – what do you do? Stop BiEst and double her progesterone (P4) until bleeding stops then go back on BiEst but keep progesterone at double.

2. After three more months you go back to standard doses and she starts bleeding again – what do you do? Get a transvaginal ultrasound[310] to check the endometrial stripe and to rule out polyps, fibroids, adenomas, or endometrial hyperplasia. If less than 5 mm then start back on BiEst/estradiol and double dose progesterone for 6 months. If stripe is > 5 mm then it might be cancerous[311] so see an Ob-Gyn as soon as possible.

Short of the referral to an Ob-Gyn another option for fibroids (leiomyomata) is Uterine Artery Embolization (UAE) which is very effective in numerous studies[312]. UAE is where these little polyvinyl alcohol balls are injected into the uterine blood vessels under radiologic guidance (it's a radiology procedure) in order to shrink the fibroids [313].

G. MALPRACTICE WARNING: ALWAYS GET (from their Ob-Gyn) or PERFORM ANNUAL PAP SMEARS[314] on each patient you have on HRT. Do not refill their prescriptions until you get the result! U.S. Preventive Services Task Force also recommends routine mammography every one to two years for women 40 years and older[315] (no upper limit) – make sure they get this, too.

H. Quick Notes on Progesterone:

  1. Expect poor absorption (except through mucosal membrane)[316].
  2. Dizziness with a high dose[317].
  3. Nipple tenderness (rare).
  4. Anxiolytic and sedative and hypnotic – good, but if a patient has this effect with their progesterone then do not use in AM with that patient[318].
  5. Oral progesterone undergoes first pass effects in liver – sublingual triturate does not[319].
  6. Side effects are usually with oral form only, not SL (sublingual).
  7. Men should not use – progesterone severely inflames vascular endothelium[320] and causes impotence!
  8. Female postmenopausal patient with insomnia? Change her progesterone to a capsule form and give the 100 mgm as Prometrium® orally at night.

I. Hargrove, JT et al from *Infertility and Reproductive Clinics of North America*[321]:
  1. Titrate progesterone to pre-menopausal levels. Give 1, 2, 3, or 4 100 mgm progesterone a day to achieve this if you need to – don't be shy. Progesterone is protective!
  2. Treat menopause as deficiency state.
  3. Correct all hormone levels that are deficient (remember: it's the hormonal milieu!).
  4. Use human micronized bio-identical hormones[322].
  5. Metabolized by normal metabolic pathways.
  6. This approach avoids problem causing metabolites.
  7. There is absolutely NO reason to not give progesterone to ALL postmenopausal women – hysterectomy or not.
  8. There is no good reason NOT to give these bio-identical estrogens and progesterone every day[323]. *Do not cycle – give them all every day.*

J. PREGNANCY PROBLEM: You have a patient on HRT and her level of progesterone comes back >100 ng/ml, why? She's pregnant until proven otherwise.

K. PMS PROBLEM: You have a pre-menopausal patient with bad PMS symptoms, what can you do? Use P4 in a 100 mgm compounded vaginal suppository for 7-14 days (prior and up to menstruation).

L. POST-PARTUM BLUES PROBLEM: You have a patient with bad post-partum depression, what can you do? Start on 100 mgm TID sublingual P4 for 7 days, then BID SL P4 for 7 days, then QD SL P4 for 7 days.

M. HOT FLASHES PROBLEM: You have a perimenopausal patient with bad hot flashes (Inhibin A in decline from the ovary is *now* felt to cause hot flashes), night sweats, and vaginal dryness -- what can you do? Start on 100 mgm TID sublingual P4 for 7 days (or until symptoms resolve) realizing they won't cycle (but who cares? Right?).

N. MIGRAINE PROBLEM: You have a perimenopausal or menopausal patient with bad migraine headaches -- what can you do? Start on 100 mgm TID to 5X DAY sublingual P4 until symptoms resolve.

O. Average age at menopause in USA? 51 years of age[324] and has an average duration of 4 years (range of 0 to 10 years).

P. UNOPPOSED CAUSES CANCER PROBLEM: Notes on endometrial hyperplasia which is generally considered a precursor to endometrial cancer. The presence of *unopposed estrogen* - which, for example, may result from exogenous estrogen therapy, anovulatory cycles, polycystic ovary syndrome (PCOS), or obesity -- has been shown to increase the likelihood of developing endometrial hyperplasia and cancer[325]. So make sure your patients are on progesterone at healthy optimized levels to prevent this from happening!

Q. The Pap test is not that helpful in identifying women who have endometrial hyperplasia -- who are at increased risk for endometrial neoplasia. In one study, the presence of normal endometrial cells in postmenopausal women not on hormonal therapy was associated with a 19 percent risk for endometrial hyperplasia or carcinoma[326].

R. OTC Natural Progesterone Creams (yam or otherwise) do NOT work, even if patients bathe in the stuff! Why? You cannot come close to getting blood levels up high enough for protection[327] (>10 ng/ml).

S. NO LIBIDO DUE TO YASMIN® PROBLEM: Final note: Yasmin® is currently the a Dr. Purser favorite birth control pill because of its very positive anti-androgenic effects. But remember those anti-androgenic effects will potentially dry up libido.

H. Human Growth Hormone (HGH or rHGH)

"r" is for recombinant which is how modern HGH is manufactured..

Twenty-four-hour growth hormone (GH) secretion reaches a peak at around puberty and by patient's early 20s has begun to decrease. Thereafter the fall in GH secretion is progressive such that by the age of 60 most adults have total 24-hour secretion rates indistinguishable from those of hypopituitary patients with organic lesions in the pituitary gland[328]. Clearly this is a valid and useful treatment for advanced sarcopenia (muscle wasting usually in the elderly)[329].

Supplementation Benefits with rHGH:

1. Improves endothelial dysfunction[330].
2. Improves Left Ventricular Hypertrophy (LVH) and Congestive Heart Failure[331] (CHF)[332].
3. Has been shown, in several studies, to decreases abdominal or visceral fat and omental fat (most critical especially in diabetes)[333].
4. Increases muscle mass[334].
5. Increases endurance (so patients can exercise a lot more)[335].
6. Mainly a healing hormone – this fact causes muscles to be less sore after work outs – decreases post-exercise recovery time[336].
7. HGH increases the very beneficial adiponectin[337] levels for cardiovascular protection.
8. WARNING: If given improperly or without the complete milieu of other critical hormones such as testosterone you can get abnormal glucose metabolism (insulin resistance)[338] (though many physicians feel this is absolutely harmless and short term in HGH replacement therapy).
9. Increases and improves rate of healing of burns[339] and surgical wounds.
10. Increases muscle mass[340].
11. Decreases and normalizes body fat with training, especially torso fat[341].
12. Sustains and improves insulin receptor and sensitivity[342].
13. Sustains and improves insulin and IGF-1 receptors and sensitivity in the brain along with being neuroprotective[343].
14. Improves thyroid resistance by improving function of the conversion receptor (with 5'-deiodinase) and peripheral thyroid retinoid receptor[344].
15. Increases endurance[345].

16. Improves immune system functionality by reversing thymic atrophy and enhancing production of T cells[346] (that's why it's so prescribed in HIV).
17. Acts as an aggressive antioxidant by stimulating superoxide dismutase[347].
18. Improves osteopenia in the elderly[348].
19. GH treatment was associated with significant improvements in total cholesterol and low-density lipoprotein[349].
20. Speeds up post-surgical healing[350] in the elderly!
21. Improves and even clears fibromyalgia symptoms[351].
22. Improves insomnia and deep REM sleep[352].
23. Can act as a neuronal rescue factor for traumatic brain injury patients with CNS injury[353].
24. Improves cognitive capabilities, memory, alertness, and motivation[354].
25. HGH readily crosses the blood brain barrier[355].
26. There is increased neuronal communication in the brain via Connexin-43 which HGH increases[356].
27. HGH improves osteopenia and osteoporosis dramatically and "GH deficient patients with osteoporosis should be considered candidates for replacement"[357].
28. HGH given to patients older than 75 years of age for hip fracture treatment caused 94% to return to pre-fracture 75%[358]. It was well tolerated.
29. A great benefit if you need it – HGH increases chondrocyte growth – very helpful for all of those elderly people with bad osteoarthritis[359].
30. HGH normalizes and shrinks intima-media thickness (possibly via NO)[360].
31. HGH improves lipid profiles, dilated cardiomyopathy and reverses atherosclerosis[361].
32. HGH reduces hsCRP levels and elevates lipoprotein(a)[362] – being very cardioprotective.
33. HGH restores thymic function and immune system functionality[363].

Time For Effect

Takes 6 months of consistent therapy to for the beneficial effects to fully take effect and kick in[364] [365]. HGH replacement works better and is more beneficial when begun at a young age[366].

Dosing and Frequency

Do not use contraband rHGH (most is fake) or secretagogues (true secretagogues work and exist but we can't get them -- for research only).

General Tips on Handling Somatropin

Handle with caution. Do not ever let get warm. Do not shake – treat like "platinum nitroglycerine." Try not to drop – remember somatropin (HGH) is a very large molecule when it exits your anterior pituitary and then it subdivides into 23 other hormones (All which assist with healing and sleep and immune function). So always handle with care. Always watch for a "bad" bottle (it probably just got too warm before use) or somatropin that gets stale (sometimes this occurs towards the end of a pen or bottle).

Norditropin® Nordiflex™ Pen (Program 120® Preferred GH):

Very high quality somatropin that seems very stable. Start with 5 mg/1.5 ml pen and have the more ill patients start at 0.1 mgm at night (4 clicks of the pen) – remember with the more ill patients (IGF-1 < 100) start low and go slow! Since they have probably not been exposed to GH for years (from pituitary damage) then they will probably have "growing pains." IT can take a year to 18 months for them to get healed.

Genotropin® MiniQuicks®:

Most expensive but does not require refrigeration so the best for travelling. Prefilled pre-jects (sterile water in one side and powdered GH in the other).

0.2 mgm is not available
0.4 mgm/day average dose

0.6 mgm/day maximum

Somatropin Secretagogues

Proof that at least one secretagogue works:

> --Hansen BS, Raun K, Nielsen KK, Johansen PB, Hansen TK, Peschke B, Lau J, Andersen PH, Ankersen M. Pharmacological characterisation of a new oral GH secretagogue, NN703. Eur J Endocrinol. 1999 Aug;141(2):180-9.

> --Raun K, Hansen BS, Johansen NL, Thogersen H, Madsen K, Ankersen M, Andersen PH. Ipamorelin, the first selective growth hormone secretagogue. Eur J Endocrinol. 1998 Nov;139(5):552-61.

> --Wren AM, Small CJ, Ward HL, Murphy KG, Dakin CL, Taheri S, Kennedy AR, Roberts GH, Morgan DG, Ghatei MA, Bloom SR. The novel hypothalamic peptide ghrelin stimulates food intake and growth hormone secretion. Endocrinology. 2000 Nov;141(11):4325-8.

Note that none of the other secretagogues work.

Levels

Females
Somatomedin-C/IGF-1 Optimal levels are 250-300 ng/mL but make sure as they near this they don't have side effects or symptoms (joint swelling, edema, etc – insulin resistance/hyperglycemia is NOT a problem).

Males
Somatomedin-C/IGF-1 Optimal levels are 300-360 ng/mL

IGFBP-3
Rarely, if ever, get this test. There is just not much need for it and it adds unnecessary cost to the lab bill.

Cost
Cost can be a major issue in the decision for your patients to take or not (these other compounded hormones are actually fairly inexpensive but rHGH is not). According to what brand and how much you take – usually $400 to $800 a month or even more.

Perceived Issues With HGH

Document Properly

Please see Appendix E for documentation advice at the end of this book.

ICU Deaths

A study was done and reported in the New England Journal of Medicine which is commonly quoted by those who have problems with giving HGH to deficient patients – this study showed an increase in mortality when ICU patients were given massive doses of HGH 16-24 IU per day when the usual adult replacement dose is only 1 IU per day. We and others believe this study was highly flawed.

> -- Takala J, Ruokonen E, Webster NR, Nielsen MS, Zandstra DF, Vundelinckx G, Hinds CJ. Increased mortality associated with growth hormone treatment in critically ill adults. N Engl J Med. 1999 Sep 9;341(11):785-92.

A key study that directly disputes this study (among hundreds of others) is:

-- Bengtsson BA, Koppeschaar HP, Abs R, Bennmarker H, Hernberg-Stahl E, Westberg B, Wilton P, Monson JP, Feldt-Rasmussen U, Wuster C. Growth hormone replacement therapy is not associated with any increase in mortality. KIMS Study Group. J Clin Endocrinol Metab. 1999 Nov;84(11):4291-2.

This shows that HGH replacement has not been associated with ANY increase in mortality in > 2000 patient years.

Cancer Deaths

We know from HIV studies that HGH improves cancer cachexia but some physicians keep connecting HGH replacement therapy with cancer causation. Here are several papers and studies that don't make those connections and their conclusions actually dispel this erroneous connection:

"No evidence of an increased risk of malignancy, recurrent or de novo."

-- Shalet SM, Brennan BM, Reddingius RE. Growth hormone therapy and malignancy. Horm Res. 1997;48 Suppl 4:29-32.

No evidence for an increased risk of tumor recurrence with HGH treatment.

-- Tacke J, Bolder U, Herrmann A, Berger G, Jauch KW. Long-term risk of gastrointestinal tumor recurrence after postoperative treatment with recombinant human growth hormone. JPEN J Parenter Enteral Nutr. 2000 May-Jun;24(3):140-4.

"NO evidence of tumor growth stimulation."

-- Fiebig HH, Dengler W, Hendriks HR. No evidence of tumor growth stimulation in human tumors in vitro following treatment with recombinant human growth hormone. Anticancer Drugs. 2000 Sep;11(8):659-64.

HGH, when given or produced endogenously, creates and elevates IGF-1 and IGF-BP3

-- Giovannucci E. Insulin-like growth factor-I and binding protein-3 and risk of cancer. Horm Res. 1999;51 Suppl 3:34-41.

IGF-1 is statistically associated with some cancers in some studies.
BUT IGF-BP3 is associated with protection against cancer.

-- Wu, et al. Inhibition of DNA Synthesis by IGFBP-3. Journal of GH and IGF Research. Oct 1999.

HGH replacement therapy is not associated with increased risk of cancer.
HGH replacement therapy is not the same as IGF.
HGH replacement therapy stimulates production of both IGF-1 and IGF-BP3.

-- Giovannucci E. Insulin-like growth factor-I and binding protein-3 and risk of cancer. Horm Res. 1999;51 Suppl 3:34-41.

And from *The Journal of Clinical Endocrinology & Metabolism* (just in case there are still any non-believers left in the audience) and the Cedars-Sinai Research Institute-University of California at Los Angeles School of Medicine, Los Angeles, California:

"Several recent compelling studies support the critical role of GH, suggesting that GH control is associated with reversal of adverse mortality rates, regardless of the nature of associated comorbidity."

"Fifteen percent of deaths in acromegaly are attributable to malignancies, which is lower than would be expected from the general population, and confirmed by Orme."

"However, *there is no clear evidence for enhanced de novo cancer initiation* in acromegaly and, as yet, no direct proven causal relationship of acromegaly with malignant disease."

 -- Melmed, S. CLINICAL PERSPECTIVE: Acromegaly and Cancer: Not a Problem? The Journal of Clinical Endocrinology & Metabolism Vol. 86, No. 7 2929-2934. Copyright © 2001 by The Endocrine Society.

Glucose Intolerance/Edema Arthralgia

These side effects only tended to occur with the older way HGH was given (low frequency high dose 2X or 3X a week). Now we know HGH should be given at a higher frequency with low dose (Example: 0.5 IU BID or IM in abdomen, rotating sites)[367].

Legal Aspects of Prescribing HGH

It is illegal to prescribe this medication for the specific diagnoses of **anti-aging needs or for body building** purposes (to enhance musculature in a young healthy individual).

"Oct. 28, 2005 — Growth hormone (GH) is illegal for off-label antiaging use, according to an article in the Oct. 26 issue of *JAMA*. This article reviews the literature concerning the uses and adverse effects of GH as well as the legal ramifications of selling, using, or prescribing it.

"Prescribing and administering GH has become a routine intervention in an industry that is variably called anti-aging, regenerative, longevity or age management medicine," lead author Thomas Perls, MD, MPH, from Boston University School of Medicine in Massachusetts, said in a news release. "Hundreds of thousands of patients who have received GH in recent years as a purported treatment for aging are unaware that they are receiving the drug illegally."

Authors of the review conclude that 1988 and 1990 amendments to the Food, Drug, and Cosmetic Act (FDCA) make off-label distribution or provision of GH to treat aging or age-related diseases illegal in the U.S. Unlike most drugs approved by the U.S. Food and Drug Administration (FDA), GH can only be distributed for indications specifically authorized by the Secretary of Health and Human Services, and these do not include aging and related disorders. In addition, the FDA has clearly indicated that GH is not a dietary supplement.

It is legal how ever to prescribe HGH for Adult HGH Deficiency – so document your reasoning well. We think this matter is so critical that we are including the entire text of health care attorney Rick Collins' recent speech at the **American Academy of Anti-Aging Medicine International Congress** in Las Vegas in 2005.

LAS VEGAS, Dec. 21 /PRNewswire/ -- Rick Collins, Esq., of the New York law firm of Collins, McDonald & Gann, P.C. (http://www.cmgesq.com), recently presented a lecture entitled "Legal Update 2005: Prescribing Growth Hormone for Adult Growth Hormone Deficiency" at the 13th Annual International Congress on Anti-Aging Medicine. The presentation clarified a commentary in the October 26, 2005 Journal of the American Medical Association entitled, "Provision or Distribution of Growth Hormone for **'Antiaging': Clinical and Legal Issues**."
    "The commentary suggests that the replacement of human growth hormone in deficient, aging adults is illegal because of a little-known federal law," said Mr. Collins, a legal authority on anabolic steroids and

performance- enhancing hormones. "But the suggestion overlooks the historical context and intent of that law."

Mr. Collins points out that the statute, part of the Anti-Drug Abuse Act of 1988, was originally written for anabolic steroids. Passed when sports doping had reached national consciousness, it was intended to combat steroid trafficking to athletes. Heightened alarm over drugs in sports, including Canadian sprinter Ben Johnson's steroid positive at the 1988 Seoul Olympics, resulted in the scheduling of anabolic steroids as controlled substances in 1990. Congress chose not to take such a drastic approach to growth hormone after testimony that growth hormone lacks the adverse psychological and physical effects of steroids. Instead, Congress took the lesser approach of inserting growth hormone into the statute that formerly applied to steroids.

"Prescribing growth hormone for non-medical reasons, including performance enhancement or 'anti-aging' in the absence of medical need, is illegal," says Mr. Collins. "But **nothing in the statute restricts physicians from treating diseases or other recognized medical conditions for which the use of growth hormone has been authorized by the FDA**. Any implication that the statute was intended to prohibit hormone replacement in mature, clinically deficient adults is incorrect."

Collins, McDonald & Gann, P.C., represents individuals and corporations on civil and criminal matters. Contact: info@cmgesq.com

Contact: Richard D. Collins, 516-294-0300, info@cmgesq.com"

Biotropin® (Canada) and Jintropin (China) are not FDA Approved and so are Illegal

On March 12, 2007 Sylvester Stallone was reported by the Reuters News Agency to have been (allegedly) arrested for importing an illegal drug – HGH (Jintropin in this case) – into Australia. Stallone apparently had 57 bottles of the Jintropin in his possession and was using it in attempt to obtain the body he had in the original Rocky© movie.

Please know that Jintropin and the Canadian Biotropin are both illegal substances especially for transport across international borders. These are NOT FDA approved and have no FDA NDC numbers. Do not import or attempt to import these substances for resale unless you want to spend time in a federal penetentiary.

I. Testosterone

Modern testosterone is now very easy in a Lipoderm® cream to supplement – just give it in compounded micronized form as an alcohol-based gel (men) or vanishing cream on labia and vaginal mucosa (women) which they rub on twice a day and is preferable. (Sublingual and oral is rapidly and extensively metabolized by the liver[368] [causing liver inflammation] and injected peaks too fast and causes too much aggression.)

Remember, this is a controlled substance (DEA) and get a DRE (digital rectal exam) and PSA (prostate specific antigen) before starting and annually thereafter[369].

Diagnosis

Hypogonadism is diagnosed easily when the usual signs and symptoms of androgen deficiency are present, or when the patient has a history of a predisposing condition such as mumps orchitis, orchiectomy, or irradiation to the pelvis or head. Conversely, the diagnosis can be more difficult in patients at an older age with less specific symptoms or an unremarkable clinical history[370] -- so document symptoms and history (see History below).

The literature advises treatment should be initiated when, in symptomatic men, levels of Free Testosterone are < 52 pg/ml or Total Testosterone levels are < 231 ng/dl[371] (but your particular lab levels may vary dramatically according to the tests they use so symptoms and history still may be more important). More importantly the Endocrine Society, through the JCEM (Journal of Clinical Endocrinology and Metabolism) and their guidelines[372]: "Testosterone Therapy in Adult Men with Androgen Deficiency Syndromes: An Endocrine Society Clinical Practice Guideline" which *advise no set* levels (though you should check both a free and total testosterone level) but only treating according to symptoms such as the following:

TABLE 1A[373]. Symptoms and signs suggestive of androgen deficiency in MEN

• Incomplete sexual development, eunuchoidism, aspermia
• Reduced sexual desire (libido) and activity
• Decreased spontaneous erections
• Breast discomfort, gynecomastia
• Loss of body (axillary and pubic) hair, reduced shaving
• Very small or shrinking testes (especially < 5 mL)
• Inability to father children, low or zero sperm counts
• Height loss, low-trauma fracture, low bone mineral density
• Reduced muscle bulk and strength
• Hot flushes, sweats

TABLE 1B[374]. Other symptoms and signs associated with androgen deficiency in MEN that are less specific than those in Table 1A

• Decreased energy, motivation, initiative, aggressiveness, self-confidence
• Feeling sad or blue, depressed mood, dysthymia
• Poor concentration and memory
• Sleep disturbance, increased sleepiness
• Mild anemia (normochromic, normocytic, in the female range)
• Increased body fat, body mass index
• Diminished physical or work performance

We advise the thorough reading of this document, also.

Testosterone History

Ask a Few Female Menopause History Questions

1. Have you suffered from vaginal dryness?
2. Have you suffered from dry uncomfortable sexual intercourse?
3. Have you suffered from red dry or inflamed vaginal tissues?
4. Have you been told you had vaginal atrophy?
5. Have you been told you had urinary incontinence such as stress incontinence or sneeze incontinence?

Benefits

What optimized testosterone levels can give your female patients:

1. Decreases endothelial resistance acting as a potent vasodilator[375].

2. Higher total testosterone and SHBG (sex hormone binding globulin) levels are inversely related to carotid atherosclerosis, suggesting their potential importance in reducing atherosclerotic risk in postmenopausal women not using HRT[376].

3. Higher free testosterone levels in men are associated with higher ejection fractions (higher cardiac output)[377].

4. Age, HDL, and **free testosterone** may be stronger predictors of degree of coronary artery disease than are blood pressure, cholesterol, diabetes, smoking, and body mass index (BMI)[378].

5. Despite the literature replete with supporting studies[379] [380], cardiologists continue to ignore the favorable benefits of natural testosterone replacement. Don't do the same.

6. There is evidence to suggest that low concentrations of testosterone are associated with an increased risk of CVD in women and men[381].

7. Testosterone concentration is inversely correlated with procoagulable factors, plasminogen activator inhibitor, and fibrinogen[382]. Give enough testosterone to obtain a good physiologic level and these coagulation factors decline.

8. Testosterone, at physiologic concentrations, induces coronary artery dilation and increases coronary blood flow in men with established coronary artery disease[383].

9. Normal physiological levels improve insulin resistance by bolstering the functionality of insulin receptors[384]. (Also, see Chapter 6 Diabetes and see Chapter 8 Alzheimer's Disease). There is an association in men between low concentrations of free and total testosterone and hyperinsulinemia[385].

10. Normal physiological levels increases muscle mass[386].

11. Lower levels predispose to increased BMI and diabetes[387].

12. Normal physiological levels prevents Alzheimer's disease. Low levels of testosterone are an independent risk factor[388]! (See Chapter 8 Alzheimer's Disease)

13. Normal physiological levels prevents osteoporosis in men and women by increasing bone mineral density (BMD)[389].

14. Normal physiological levels improves erectile dysfunction in men[390].

15. Normal physiological levels improves libido and well-being in men and women (in women who have undergone oophorectomy and hysterectomy, transdermal testosterone improves sexual function and psychological well-being[391] *[Author-- as reported in the New England Journal of Medicine using optimized levels from younger women who were menstruating, confirming once again our repeated observation that the peer reviewed studies use the optimized levels and so should the practitioners]*).

16. In adult males, testosterone maintains muscle mass and strength, fat distribution, bone mass, erythropoiesis, male hair pattern, libido and potency, and spermatogenesis[392].

17. Testosterone increases HGH production in the elderly -- it is critical to create that rich hormonal milieu or stew that allows all eight cylinders of your patient's hormone engines to fire properly. In light of a Mayo Clinic study having shown that giving hypogonadal men, especially elderly men, testosterone causes them to also increase production of endogenous HGH[393]. This is awesome and a heck of a lot cheaper then giving rHGH!

18. 35% of heart patients treated with testosterone *improved* by at least one NYHA (New York Heart Association) class[394].

19. Testosterone replacement therapy improves functional capacity and symptoms in men with moderately severe heart failure[395]. *[Why don't cardiologists put all of their patients on this?]*

20. Testosterone can dramatically improve endurance especially in the frail elderly[396] (but really since it will build muscle and bone mass this can occur at almost any level from age 40 years on[397]).

21. Sex hormones play a key role in numerous physiologic processes and functions and clearly impact wound healing in the all ages of patients[398] but especially the elderly[399].

22. Maintaining appropriate levels until death allows improved cognition, better affect, more rapid thinking/processing skills[400] and decision making and better muscle mass[401].

23. With your erectile dysfunction patients don't ever give Viagra® until you have worked them up for hypogonadism or testosterone deficiency[402]. Experience shows you will often need to give both testosterone[403] and sildenafil (or your favorite phosphodiesterase inhibitor) to more adequately treat some ED cases.

24. Testosterone in patients can not only improve insulin resistance but increase the number and health of insulin receptors[404]. First, the lack of testosterone in men has been strongly associated with metabolic syndrome[405]. Second, giving testosterone to these men can help clear up the insulin resistance and absolve the pre-diabetic stage[406].

25. Testosterone improves vascular resistance, reduces systolic blood pressure[407], improves dyslipidemias[408] (lowers triglycerides, raises HDL), and improves cardiac output.

26. Normal physiological levels causes improvement in osteoporosis[409] as is clear in a number of studies[410].

27. Testosterone in hypogonadal men improves Alzheimer's disease (see Alzheimer's Chapter), Multiple Sclerosis (MS)[411], Huntington's disease[412], Parkinson's disease, and others. As a matter of fact, testosterone loss may be a risk factor for cognitive decline and possibly for dementia[413] and is clearly neuroprotective[414] and exogenous supplementation proved beneficial for cognitive and brain function in elderly men.

28. Testosterone supplementation can increase red blood cells, an extremely beneficial factor for most older men *and women*, causing a relative erythrocytosis. Do not be mistaken – this is not a polycythemia nor a polycythemia vera (see below) – this is just a beneficial eyrthrocytosis that deserves no treatment, and even minimal observation[415]. Most men *and women* who are hypogonadal are also anemic[416] and supplementing them with testosterone can often resolve this.

29. Testosterone replacement therapy (TRT) improves lower urinary tract symptoms in men (LUTS – urinary frequency, urgency, halting or residual urine in the bladder, etc) and shrinks BPH. Erectile dysfunction (ED), which is absolutely associated with hypogonadisim or low levels of testosterone, has now been associated with LUTS[417] and BPH[418].

30. In women, testosterone is the main hormone that prevents urogenital and vaginal atrophy – save your female patients from decades of dry vaginas, poor sex lives and embarrassing stress incontinence by giving them a little testosterone just like their ovaries did!

31. Testosterone decline with aging in men is associated with osteoarthritis development[419] and worsening rheumatoid arthritis[420].

32. Testosterone Replacement Therapy (TRT), unlike what is commonly believed, is NOT associated with causing frank PIN (prostate intraepithelial neoplasia) to become full prostate cancer. After 1 year of TRT men with PIN treated at Beth Israel Deaconess Medical Center at the Harvard Medical School do NOT have a greater increase in PSA or a significantly increased risk of cancer than men without PIN. These results indicate that TRT is not contraindicated in men with a history of PIN[421].

33. Contrary to what your local cardiologist says (and some papers erroneously claim as a side effect) physiological testosterone replacement did not adversely affect blood coagulation status

(plasminogen activator inhibitor-1 (PAI-1), fibrinogen, tissue plasminogen activator (tPA) and full blood count)[422].

34. Low levels of testosterone in elderly men increase fall risk by 40%[423] (probably secondary to weaker antigravity and balance muscles). Fall risk was higher in men with lower bioavailable testosterone levels. The effect of testosterone level was independent of poorer physical performance, suggesting that the effect of testosterone on fall risk may be mediated by other androgen actions.

Dose

Younger Women (<50 y.o.): 20 mgm/gram in vanishing cream – start with ¼ gram at night on inner arms (if poor results you can advance to inner thighs or the vaginal mucosa). (For women describe it as a chocolate chip sized amount on vaginal lips and mucosa.)

Older Women (>50 y.o.): 30 mgm/gram in vanishing cream – start with ¼ gram at night on inner arms (if poor results you can advance to inner thighs or the vaginal mucosa). (For women describe it as a chocolate chip sized amount on vaginal lips and mucosa.)

Levels

Men with hypogonadotropic hypogonadism have low plasma testosterone levels and luteinizing hormone levels that may be low or low-normal. When borderline total testosterone values are found, or the clinical picture and the serum testosterone levels disagree, additional measures of circulating androgens are needed. The most accurate indicator of hypogonadism is the concentration of testosterone that is not bound to sex hormone binding globulin (the concentration of bioavailable testosterone or Free Testosterone)[424].

This can be problematic because labs change. The two most common types of labs would be Quest-based numbers or LabCor-based numbers.

The Andrology Society in their position statement[425] feels that a morning Total Testosterone level below 300 ng/dL using a reliable *assay from a good laboratory*[426] is necessary for the diagnosis.

Female
Quest®
Treated Optimized Free Testosterone should be 8.0 -10 ng/mL or slightly greater
Or
NON-QUEST® labs (LabCor®)
Treated Optimized Free Testosterone level of 3.8-4.0 pg/ml or slightly greater.

Male
Quest ®
Total Testosterone (treated) should be near 1000 ng/mL
Free Testosterone Optimal Range 30-40 pg/dL – get the levels to around 40 pg/dl.
or
NON-QUEST labs (LabCor®)
Free Testosterone 180-210 ng/dL – get the levels to around 210 ng/dl.

Potential Side Effects – Explanations or Treatments

1. Prostate enlargement (misunderstood) – from increased DHT. Give finasteride (Proscar®) or dutasteride (Avodart®).
2. Hair loss – give spironolactone 100 mgm a day to men or women
3. Hair growth/hirsutism -- give spironolactone 100 mgm a day to men or women
4. Acne – rare except with injectable in men (DO NOT USE) and when women have really high levels.

5. Prostate cancer? Literature does not really support[427] – find it if you can[428]…
6. Increased libido – problematic if older spouse (with chronic dyspareunia, etc) is not on testosterone, too. Can cause divorce. Warn them.
7. Aggression – usually only with injectable testosterone
8. Decreased sperm production – more common with injectable
9. Erythrocytosis is NOT Polycythemia – often stated erroneously as such but is not and is almost always just a healthy erythrocytosis. Look at diagnostic lab requirements of PV then decide[429] [430].
10. Fluid retention -- give spironolactone 100 mgm a day to men or women
11. Gynecomastia – give Arimidex 0.5mgm twice a week.
12. Decreased testicular size—from decreased LH/FSH in men.
13. Super high Total Testosterone level (1200 or 1450 or thereabouts?) and normal or optimized Free Testosterone? Then you have high Sex Hormone Binding Globulin (SHBG).
14. SHBG synthesis is stimulated by estrogens and decreased by androgens and obesity[431]. Think aromatase inhibitor if your males patient has super high total testosterone and gynecomastia (one of the rare times to use Arimidex®).
15. Infertility -- TESTOSTERONE WARNING: If your patient wishes to maintain Leydig cell functionality and fertility, give 2000-5000 units of injectable β-HCG each week[432]:
    A. No decreases in testicular size.
    B. No decreases in sperm count.
    C. Younger men remain fertile.

More About "Polycythemia" Seen With Testosterone Replacement

This is by definition NOT a true polycythemia as there is not a "poly-" component – multiple cell line elevations (platelets, RBCs and WBCs) – the only cell elevated with these patients is the RBC. If anything else is elevated then you might indeed have a true polycythemia *unrelated* to the giving of testosterone – and this should be evaluated appropriately. This is by definition only an idiopathic erythrocytosis.

e·ryth·ro·cy·to·sis (-rthr-s-tss) n.
An abnormal increase in the number of circulating red blood cells.

--The American Heritage® Stedman's Medical Dictionary, 2nd Edition Copyright © 2004 by Houghton Mifflin Company. Published by Houghton Mifflin Company. All rights reserved.

There is no JAK2 kinase (V617F) mutation associated with these patients (as it is usually with a true polycythemia vera) and their hematocrit is rarely elevated above 56 or 58 %. This is also, according to expert hematologists, a "stable disease with a low thrombotic risk and a low, if any, tendency to spontaneous progression to acute leukemia or myelofibrosis," with no treatments necessary[433].

Please be aware that numerous articles on testosterone oddly (and erroneously) state that testosterone supplementation can cause polycythemia[434] or polycythemia vera and supplementation could be problematic because of this or should be stopped if this occurs. Yet when one digs further into the references of these articles the same odd error tends to repeat itself without validation.

Just know that replacement with reasonable amounts of testosterone is known to be not only very safe[435] but highly beneficial.

Blood Dyscrasia ≠ Idiopathic Erythrocytosis ≠ Polycythemia Vera

Increasing Aromatase Activity?

Aromatase converts the testosterone you are giving to estrogen— usually not a good thing. These are things that increase aromatase activity:

3. Genetics
4. Excess testosterone – injections
5. ETOH (alcohol)
6. Obesity
7. Diuretics
8. Vitamin C Deficiency
9. Low Soy Diet
10. Grapefruit

Avoiding Aromatization

Aromatization is where testosterone is converted within the human body to estrogen – feminizing the man (usually minimally), causing gynecomastia, increased abdominal adipose, and erectile dysfunction.

Advise exercising first (1-4-7 and weight lifting. This is a viable along with, of course, reducing their testosterone dose.

Anastrozole (Arimidex®) is the aromatase inhibitor of choice. The drug is appropriately used when using substantial amounts of aromatizing steroids, or when one is prone to gynecomastia. Arimidex® does not have the side effects of other aromatase inhibitors and can achieve a high degree of estrogen blockade. Keep in mind anastrozole is very expensive.

So reducing the dose of testosterone you're prescribing and having them exercise more is *a much cheaper option* than Arimidex®. Also and most critically it is just about never really needed but if you must prescribe Arimidex® give 0.5 mgm orally twice a week.

Does Testosterone Elevate Liver Enzymes?

Some times the side effect of the elevation of liver enzymes is also noted as a side effect with testosterone replacement therapy. This may rarely occur with the higher doses of the injectable testosterone cypionate (though even this is not supported by any literature searches) but is not seen with the topical cream version.

So if your patient's LFTs jump be aware that it is probably something else.

Does Testosterone Replacement Therapy Really Cause Prostate Cancer?

Though testosterone replacement was widely accepted in the past to cause prostate cancer (and is still by some urologists and most attorneys) it is becoming more and more clear in the recent literature that just the opposite is true – low levels of testosterone (like most older men have when they usually tend to develop prostate cancer) appear instead to be associated with prostate cancers[436][437].

Low Serum Testosterone Levels = Higher Risk To Form Prostate Cancer

Actually, there is currently no evidence that testosterone replacement can promote a *de novo* or pre-existing prostatic malignancy in hypogonadal men[438] and there are strong indications that normal testosterone levels play a protective role in the causation of prostate cancer.

MALPRACTICE WARNING: Have patients sign a release/informed consent if they wish to take testosterone and are at high risk for breast cancer or prostate cancer.

MALPRACTICE WARNING: If testosterone levels are oddly too low prior to treatment, then get a PROLACTIN LEVEL to rule out a pituitary adenoma[439] (prolactinomas account for most elevations of prolactin level higher than 100 μg/L; serum prolactin levels greater than 200 μg/L almost invariably indicate a prolactinoma).

MALPRACTICE WARNING: Prior to starting testosterone in males obtain a PSA and do a digital rectal exam (DRE). Follow these regularly – re-check every year. Do not renew prescriptions without obtaining annually and having in chart. Studies have not absolutely confirmed the association of exogenous testosterone with prostate cancer[440] (if anything as noted above the opposite has occurred) but be safe and check for PSA changes any way[441].

Notes About Dihydroepiandrostenedione (DHT)

DHT is 10-15% of total testosterone
Levels – Normal 50-100
Levels with testosterone? 100-500
Good effects on libido
Does not convert to estrogen
Does not effect prostate (contrary to popular beliefs – not supported)
Approved in gel form
Bad effects on hair loss
> D. Give finasteride (Propecia®) 1 mgm twice a week – decreases serum DHT
> E. Saw Palmetto does not really work, only decreases intraprostatic binding of testosterone, estrogen and DHT.

PSA Discussion[442]

Normal PSA   < 4.0

Abnormal PSA > 4.0 → Measure Total PSA if > 2.5 → Free PSA
                                        <10% → CANCER *****
                                        10-20% → INDETERMINATE
                                        >20% → NO CANCER

Who Needs Further Testing?

If your patient's tests come back abnormal or kind of abnormal (borderline) you have other options:
Urology Consult
Prostatic Ultrasound
12 Sample Needle Biopsy

J. Cortisol

One theory for the hypothalamus loss of regulation is that it is damaged by the hormone *cortisol*. Cortisol is produced from the *adrenal glands* (located on the kidneys) and cortisol is considered to be a dark-hormone caused by and responsible for stress.

Cortisol:

Increases as we age.
Causes diabetes through weight gain[443].
Suppresses immune system functionality.
Worsens glucose intolerance, causes hypertension and other medical problems[444].
Worsens cardiac risk and CVD[445].
Ratio lowers with melatonin which is beneficial.

J. Alcohol and Narcotic Abuse

People who abuse or heavily use alcohol and narcotics tend to wipe out their hormone levels – mostly lowering testosterone levels to zero. These people (especially the men) are often totally hypogonadal and have no libido (think these patients definitely need testosterone supplementation when you see them)[446].

K. Lab Error

There is a lot of lab error out there. If you get lab numbers that seem really out of line with treatment and clinical reality then repeat the lab. Use your brain and reason to clarify any issues you have with odd lab numbers.

L. More OTC Nutriceuticals

Vitamin D – The Lost Vitamin/Lost Steroid Hormone

Vitamin D is a critical part of this entire prevention concept. Technically it is NOT a vitamin but a steroid hormone which could also explain some of its powerful benefits. Most people in colder climates are vitamin D deficient (levels below 25-30 nmol/L) especially if they are of dark skin national heritage (African American, Hispanic, Eastern Indian or Asian[447]). Older patients, especially in nursing homes, rarely get enough sunlight, and even those who might, do not have the skin capacity to properly absorb and convert the appropriate amounts of Vitamin D to aide them – that's why 82% + have levels that are too low[448] – this is because Vitamin D2 is converted in the skin to the most active form, D3.

Signs and Symptoms

Patients with optimized Vitamin D levels absorb about 30% of their gut calcium. With really low level of Vitamin D this drops to 15% or less, and parathyroid hormone (PTH) increases in an attempt to maintain cellular calcium levels, pulling calcium from the bones (where it is theoretically in storage) causing osteopenia or even osteoporosis.

Patients with severe vitamin D deficiency and hypocalcemia present with classic findings of neuromuscular irritability, including numbness, paresthesias, muscle cramps, laryngospasm, Chvostek's sign, Trousseau's phenomenon, tetany, and seizures[449].

Chvostek's Sign

Refers to an abnormal reaction to the stimulation of the facial nerve. When the facial nerve is tapped at the angle of the jaw, the facial muscles on the same side of the face will contract momentarily (typically a twitch of the nose or lips) because of hypocalcemia or hypomagnesia and hyperexcitability of nerves[450].

Trousseau's Sign (of latent tetany)

In a patient with hypocalcaemia, carpal spasm may be elicited by occluding the brachial artery. To perform the maneuver, a blood pressure cuff is placed around the arm and inflated to a pressure greater than the systolic blood pressure and held in place for 3 minutes. If carpal spasm occurs, manifested as flexion at the wrist and metacarpophalangeal joints, extension of the distal interphalangeal and proximal interphalangeal joints, and adduction of the thumb and fingers, the sign is said to be positive and the patient likely has hypocalcemia. This sign may become positive before other gross manifestations of hypocalcemia such as hyperreflexia and tetany, but is generally believed to be less sensitive than Chvostek's sign for hypocalcemia[451].

Disease States

The adult patient with severe vitamin D depletion develops osteomalacia and presents with localized bone pain, antigravity muscle weakness, difficulty rising from a chair or walking, and pseudofractures[452].

Other disease states and characteristics associated with the development of vitamin D deficiency include significant renal or hepatic disease, history of gastric resection or bypass, malabsorption, and use of certain medications such as anticonvulsants[453].

Benefits

Vitamin D is a powerful PROHORMONE which helps patients absorb calcium from the small bowel into their systems for an appropriate increase bone mineral density (BMD). It is the Vitamin D3 that affects the BMD by stopping osteoclast activity (which remove the calcium from the bone) and only slightly increasing calcium deposition into the bone matrix[454]. Along with the sex hormones, estrogen and/or testosterone, with which it works synergistically, Vitamin D does a better job (and very naturally so) especially when given with Vitamin K, these substances aggressively rebuild bone, unlike ANTHING else on the market and are far more beneficial overall for patients.

MALPRACTICE WARNING: Do not start anyone on osteoporosis therapies without FIRST checking a serum 25(OH)D level.

1. Appropriate Vitamin D levels reduces essential hypertension[455] and associated inflammation, reducing the risk of CVD[456].

2. Because of #1 (above), Vitamin D clearly and effectively decreases osteoporosis and increases bone mineral density (BMD)[457]. *[In this study quoted levels are on average 115 nmol/L and these were just people suntanning and without side effects or toxicity from that high Vitamin D level.]*

3. Appropriate Vitamin D levels drastically reduce endothelial dysfunction and inflammation[458], reducing the risk of CVD[459].

4. Appropriate Vitamin D levels will also strengthen muscles in those who have low levels[460], especially the *frail* elderly, and protects against falls[461], thus protecting against one of the most common causes of death in the elderly! Studies have shown that patients in nursing homes with good levels (we believe this to be 90-100 nmol/L) have nearly 50-65%[462] reduction in fall risks[463]!

5. Appropriate Vitamin D levels can also improve postural balance in the elderly[464]. (That little old lady stuck in a wheelchair over in the corner because she's too weak to walk? Try getting her Vitamin D levels up and stand back to watch what happens!) As a matter of fact, low 25(OH)D levels can increase a patient's risk that they will be forced into considering admission to a nursing home[465]!

6. Appropriate Vitamin D levels (95-100 nmol/L) will also protect against breast cancer and recurrence of breast cancer[466]. We know from another study[467] that having appropriate levels of Vitamin D can actually potentially lower your patient's risk by 27% or more.

7. Appropriate Vitamin D levels will strongly protect against colorectal cancer and recurrence of colorectal cancer[468]. Patient's in the lowest half of the 25(OH)D levels of women measured had, on average, a 2.52 overall risk (152 % increase)!

8. Appropriate Vitamin D levels will also protect against ovarian cancer and recurrence of ovarian cancer[469].

9. Appropriate Vitamin D levels will also protect against pancreatic cancer and recurrence[470].

10. From a recent study at Harvard[471] we know now that appropriate Vitamin D levels (90+ nmol/L) can reduce the symptoms of MS (multiple sclerosis) dramatically and totally resolve the symptoms in some patients, *especially if addressed prior to age 20.* In some countries where there is bright daily sunlight and very warm weather, MS is almost non-existent (India for example where it so uncommon that any cases get a mention in the literature[472]) – could this be because they almost never have members of their population with low Vitamin D levels?

11. Low Vitamin D levels are found in the majority of more ill Type 2 diabetics, also[473]. Could the insulin receptor failure (i.e. insulin resistance) be related to the endothelial dysfunction and inflammation caused by the lack of this anti-inflammatory steroid hormone? *[Also, in the study quoted the cutoff levels used, we believe, were very low and the percentage would have been higher if more realistic levels had been considered.]*

12. Appropriate Vitamin D levels (32-40 ng per mL [95-100 nmol/L]) can reduce the symptoms and even reduce the risk of developing of SLE (systemic lupus erythematosus), especially among African Americans females[474].

13. Appropriate Vitamin D levels (95-100 nmol/L) can reduce the symptoms and even reduce the risk of developing of schizophrenia and or acute psychosis[475].

14. Vitamin D insufficiency is present in almost all CHF patients[476]m improving when their levels are optimized.

15. Low Vitamin D levels are positively associated with obesity (BMI > 30) and obese patients, as suggested by one of the leading researchers in Vitamin D research, should be checked for deficiency[477].

16. Vitamin D deficiency has been associated in a number of studies with fibromyalgia[478].

17. The current recommendations for the upper limits of what dose is safe in adults should be 10X what is stated. 10,000 Units of Vitamin D2 a day is probably within the safe dose for almost adults[479]! 10,000 Units!

Pricing

All these benefits and for only a few pennies a day? That's the best advice in this book.

Vitamin D Levels

Vitamin D levels are covered by Medicare in certain situations but are not cheap -- $150 on average but as you can se from above are well worth obtaining.

0-15 ng per mL (25-32 nmol/L) is too low.

16-20 ng per mL (40-50 nmol/L up to 75 nmol/L) as some of the literature suggests, is probably not high enough – NO MATTER YOUR LABORATORY norms!

32-40 ng per mL (80-95-100 nmol/L is about where levels should be and not above 100 nmol/L.

Vitamin D Dosing

Vitamin D3, as we've said, is dirt cheap. Know that D3 (cholecalciferol) is about three times (3X) more potent than D2 (ergocalciferol)[480]. Also, 30 to 120 minutes of sunlight will usually give 20,000 units of Vitamin D3 to your younger patients. Plus, most experts believe the UVB (and incidentally UVA) exposure to increase melanoma risk is too great to achieve proper Vitamin D levels[481] so it's best to obtain appropriate levels.

Start with 50,000 IU of compounded Vitamin D2 (ergocalciferol) orally a week for 8 weeks (some physicians just give that dose daily for eight days). Then, *at a minimum*, you should give 1,000 IU of Vitamin D3 (cholecalciferol) a day thereafter[482].

Realistically most patients will need 2,000 IU a day or more (3,000 IU) to get and keep their levels up into the 50-80 nmol/L range [483] (which we believe is not high enough) and some nursing home patients and breast cancer survivors may need as much as 8,000 IU per day to protect them by getting them into the appropriate range (very near 100 nmol/L).

Unlike what used to be believed, it is VERY difficult to obtain toxic levels or to get toxic on Vitamin D but if in doubt check levels (25(OH)D)[484].

Side Effects and Problems

MALPRACTICE WARNING: Unexpected very low calcium and 25(OH)D levels (i.e. in a young active person) should lead you to obtain a serum PTH level to rule out a parathyroid tumor[485].

L-Arginine

Rule: Always Take L-Arginine When You Take Testosterone

L-Arginine supercharges androgens, multiplying the beneficial results you gain by testosterone supplementation.

Benefits:

1. Increases Muscle Development and Strength[486]
2. Improves Angina[487] [488] and Dyslipidemia[489]
3. Improves Hypertension[490]
4. Acts as a Potent Antioxidant[491]
5. Can Improve Oligospermia[492]
6. Enhances Endurance[493] (exercise tolerance especially in heart failure patients).
7. Mainly for men (or women with heart disease) -- take 1 gram of L-Arginine a day (your patients can go up to two a day).
8. Assists in lowering cholesterol so it's cardioprotective[494].
9. Assists in elevating sperm counts and motility so it helps in sexual dysfunction (via the beneficial nitric oxide pathway) and sometime in male infertility issues[495].
10. Diets with adequate L-arginine boosts IGF-1 levels[496].

Acetyl-L-Carnitine

Acetyl-l-carnitine has been shown to improve neurological function[497] even after we stop taking it, suggesting that acetyl-l-carnitine may re-program neuronal and neurotransmitter functions to enable the brain to function in a more youthful, energetic state. Acetyl-l-carnitine is also beneficial to heart muscle cells, immune function and probably enhances energy production in every cell of the body. The multi-faceted benefits of acetyl-l-carnitine in brain cells makes it the single most important supplement we can take to maintain and improve overall neurological function.

As previously discussed in the cardiovascular chapter (Chapter 1) carnitine is an amino acid derivative that is found in all cells of the body, especially striated muscles. It is synthesized in the liver, kidneys, and brain from the amino acids lysine and methionine. Two analogs of carnitine, acetyl-L-carnitine and propionyl-L-carnitine, have been used clinically. And carnitine plays an important role in the transport of free fatty acids across the inner mitochondrial membranes for energy production. It is a cofactor in carbohydrate metabolism and has been noted to reduce the buildup of toxic metabolites in an ischemic condition. And it is widely utilized by patients with a variety of cardiovascular conditions

L-Theanine

The neuroprotective effects of theanine and catechins contained in green tea are well known and supported in the literature[498]. L-theanine offers several neuroprotective actions.

Wiley Protocol

Suzanne Somers touts this in her most recent book. We do not believe this overcomplicated regimen works, the major problem being about massive doses of progesterone (8,200 mg a month when the average female should get about 3,000 mg a month). We only refer you to two websites to counter all the of the misinformation and requests we seem to get for this protocol

http://www.rhythmicliving.org/rhythmicliving/home.html or wileywatch.org

ALL LEVELS – PROGRAM 120®
CHEAT SHEET

Hormones	**Optimized Levels**
DHEAS	
Males	500-660 µg/dL
Females	200-250 µg/dL
Free T3	3.0-4.0 pg/mL
Estradiol	
NEWLY menopausal	75-100 pg/mL
OLDER menopausal	>50 pg/mL .
Progesterone	>10 ng/mL < 20 ng/ml)
Testosterone	
Females	
Quest® Lab	
Free Testosterone	8.0 -10 ng/mL
NON-QUEST labs (LabCor®)	
Free Testosterone	3.8-4.0 pg/ml
Males	
Quest® Lab	
Total Testosterone	800-1200 ng/mL
Free Testosterone	30-40 pg/dL
NON-QUEST labs (LabCor®)	
Free Testosterone	180-210 ng/dL
HGH	
Females	
Somatomedin-C/IGF-1	250-300 ng/mL
Males	
Somatomedin-C/IGF-1	300-360 ng/mL

The Program 120® Checklist

- ☐ Get a complete risk and hormone lab profile performed at your physician's office *[+5-10 (yrs) or more!]*
- ☐ No matter who you are, obtain a 25(OH)D level to check your Vitamin D level. If not optimized (close to 100) get it there by taking 1000, 2000 or even 3000 IU a day of Vitamin D3 orally until optimized *[+5-10 (yrs) or more!]*
- ☐ If you are MALE make sure you check IGF-1 level, total and free testosterone levels, DHEA level, TSH, free T4, and especially a free T3 (harder to get because most labs won't do it and doctors won't order it), a PSA level, and a complete lipid profile. *[+5-10 (yrs) or more!]*
- ☐ If you are FEMALE make sure you check IGF-1 level, total and free testosterone levels, DHEA level, TSH, free T4, and especially a free T3 (harder to get because most labs won't do it and doctors won't order it), an estradiol level, progesterone level and a complete lipid profile. *[+5-10]*
- ☐ Get on an appropriate dose of timed release micronized melatonin (refer to our chapter on HRT) – you must titrate it according to the hangover or lack thereof the next morning. *[+5]*
- ☐ If you are younger than about 51 and female and wish to maintain tes levels take injectable HCG 300-500 units per week. *[+15-20 (yrs) or more!]*
- ☐ If you are older than 40 and female get on a micronized timed release DHEA supplement (10 mgm - 25 mgm a day). *[+15-20 (yrs) or more!]*

- [ ] If you are older than 40 and have a history of any traumatic brain trauma or a family history of Alzheimer's disease get on a micronized timed release pregnenolone supplement (100 mgm a day). *[+5-10 (yrs) or more!]*
- [ ] If you have any symptoms of hypothyroidism (fatigue, coldness, dyslipidemia, etc) or abnormal TSH or T3 or T4 level get on a dessicated mixed thyroid supplement capsule (60 mgm - 240 mgm/1 grain to 4 grains a day average dose). *[+15-20 (yrs) or more!]*
- [ ] To elevate your hormones (especially HGH and testosterone) exercise at a moderate level at least one hour a day. *[+15-20 (yrs) or more!]*
- [ ] Get your BMI below 25 ASAP. *[+15-20 (yrs) or more!]*
- [ ] If your levels are not optimal, whether male or female, add a testosterone supplement to your regimen until your levels are properly optimized. *[+15-20 (yrs) or more!]*
- [ ] If you are female and postmenopausal add estrogen (biologically identical human hormone BiEst) human progesterone, and testosterone to your regimen. Follow closely and get your levels optimized. *[+15-20 (yrs) or more!]*
- [ ] If you have had your uterus and ovaries removed (no matter what age) take everything – BiEst, Testosterone, DHEA, Progesterone. Save your life! *[+20-25 (yrs) or more!][Do NOT TAKE DHEA though if you have a breast cancer family or personal risk factor.]*
- [ ] If you are older female and have any of the 5 Bs or signs of estrogen dominance get on human progesterone supplementation (100 mgm - 400 mgm a day sublingual triturate(s)). *[+15-20 (yrs) or more!]*
- [ ] Avoid alcoholic beverages because they can decrease testosterone levels. *[+15-20 (yrs) or more!]*
- [ ] FEMALES: Get annual Pap smear and annual mammograms especially if you are on hormone replacement therapy (HRT). *[+5-10 (yrs) or more!]*
- [ ] MALES: Get annual digital rectal exam and PSA lab exam. *[+5-10]*
- [ ] If you are on testosterone add L-arginine at 1000 mgm a day as a supplement. *[+5-10]*
- [ ] If you are at risk for viral illnesses or have shingles add Thymus Protein Boost A® (to boost your T cell functionality) to your regimen (one packet twice a week up to one packet a day). *[+5-10]*

Other Problems We Address

Chapter 12
Sexual Health

In the United States, 91% of married adult men and 84% of married adult women consider it important to have a satisfying sex life[499].

The prevalence of sexual dysfunction increases as men and women age; about 40-45% of *all* adult women and 20-30% of *all* adult men have at least one manifest sexual dysfunction. Common risk factor categories associated with sexual dysfunction exist for men and women including: individual general health status, diabetes mellitus, cardiovascular disease, other genitourinary disease, psychiatric/psychological disorders, other chronic diseases, and socio-demographic conditions[500].

Overall Causes of ED (from above)

Vascular Causes	50-56%
Psychological Causes	20-33%
Pharmacologic Causes	6-8%
Operative Causes	6-8%
Neurologic Causes	3-4%
Endocrinologic Causes	2-3%
Traumatic	1%

The Program 120® team feels that the vascular causes are mostly associated with a decline in testosterone levels (hypogonadism is strongly associated with vascular and insulin resistance which causes endothelial damage) – this is not a unique position[501].

The Program 120® Checklist

☐ Lose weight – you've been prescribed **The 11 Step Program 120® Eating Plan** to follow – do it – you will not be hungry. *[+15-20]*

☐ Consistently reduce your calories by 500 Kcal a day. *[+5-10 (yrs) or more!]*

☐ If you are at low risk get approved for exercise by your physician (focusing on your heart) prior to starting the exercise program. *[+25-30 (yrs) or more!]*

☐ If you're older then 40 or have any cardiovascular risk factors get cIMT and hsCRP levels to assess your risk prior to starting an exercise program. *[+10-15 (yrs) or more!]*

☐ Get your IGF-1 level checked to see if HGH would be of benefit. *[+5-10 (yrs) or more!]*

☐ Whether young or middle aged exercise at least 30 minutes a day 6 days a week (ideally and hour or more a day 6 gays a week) *[+20-25 (yrs) or more!]*

☐ Get your serum free testosterone level checked to see if it would be of benefit. *[+10-15 (yrs) or more!]*

☐ Get your TSH, free T4, free T3 checked to se if thyroid would be of benefit. *[+10-15 (yrs) or more!]*

☐ Take a topical human biologically identical testosterone cream or gel. *[+25-30 (yrs) or more!]*

☐ Add L-arginine to your diet through a quality supplement of 1000-4000 mgm a day. *[+15-20 (yrs) or more!]*

☐ Add fish oil capsules three times a day to your regimen. *[+10-15 (yrs) or more!]*

☐ Exercise some more – weight lifting causes the release of serum testosterone. *[+5-10 (yrs) or more!]*

☐ If you have hypertension, control your blood pressure with an ARB such as telmisartan. *[+15-20 (yrs) or more!]*

☐ Reduce your vascular inflammation such as hs-CRP levels by controlling your cardiovascular risk factors (Chapter 1). *[+10-15 (yrs) or more!]*

☐ Always wear proper protection! *[+15-20 (yrs) or more!]*

Chapter 13
The Program 120® Proper
Eating & Lifestyle Modifications

Classification of Obesity

In the United States, 64% of adults are now overweight or obese[502], and the numbers are projected to climb dramatically in the future. The World Health Organization has a formula for obesity as follows:

Body Mass Index = kg/m2

The World Health Organization (WHO) defines a body mass index (BMI) as the weight in kilograms divided by the square of the height in meters (kg/m2). Also the WHO has defined a BMI over 25 kg/m2 as being overweight, and a BMI of over 30 kg/m2 as obese[503].

Exercise

Exercise Pre-Screening

For screening remember that a simple EKG is not enough – and an exercise treadmill test (ETT) is no longer the standard[504] – why? The American Heart Association is now strongly discouraging the use of ETT as a screening tool because if the patient is asymptomatic they have <1% chance in a year of having a heart attack and their coronary artery must be at least 70% occluded to provide a positive ETT result – this is not sufficient. Instead from the Atherosclerosis Risk in Communities (ARIC) study we know we should order a Carotid Intima-Media Thickness (cIMT) test[505]. This test is highly predictive of serious silent cardiovascular disease and is the now the standard.

More recently the Before starting to exercise, according the Screening for Heart Attack Prevention and Education (SHAPE) Task Force[506], even your asymptomatic adults should be screened with noninvasive tests for heart disease in order to protect themselves (and yourself). According to SHAPE a cIMT or 64-slice CT scan[507] would be most appropriate. At Program 120® we believe, if available, the 64 slice CT scan is the most preferable and a great new non-invasive way to look perform "angiography" (also called ECG-Gated 64-MDCT Angiography)[508].

MALPRACTICE WARNING: Do not just get an Exercise Stress Test (EST) to screen – this won't be positive until anterior descending coronary artery is 70-80% occluded.

Exercise That Really Works

Again we need to keep this simple. If they can walk and if they're financially able, encourage your patient to buy a treadmill and buy the best one they can afford.

So why a higher-end treadmill?

Your patients can use them at home where it's safe, where there are no obstacles, where there is no ice and no slipping, no risk of getting mugged, minimal pollution, no traffic to run them over, where a bathroom is near for potty breaks, where water is near if they get thirsty, and where help is near if they need it. Plus, nothing is worse than your patients working out and getting in better and better shape and then having this nice treadmill they bought break down or the motor go bad or the platform you run on crack or go bad (happens often with less expensive treadmills) – so there's a method to our madness.

What are the best treadmills? Your patients should use a professional model if they can find it. One with a weight limit to match their body size – there are 350 pound treadmills out there. Woodway™, Nautilus™, NordicTrack™ (8600 only), LifeFitness™, Precor™ and Landice™ (comes with a real serious lifetime warranty) all make high end, high quality treadmills which would be excellent choices for patients and physicians alike.

Please refer to the Program 120® website for assistance in finding the best treadmill – currently we believe it to be just about any Landice® model as they come with a lifetime (and we mean lifetime) warranty. When your patients buy a Landice® treadmill, they will be able to use it forever just make sure they maintain it with a proper maintenance kit and have it set up correctly.

A set of free weights is also very handy for light weight before or after a work out on the treadmill.

If hips or back or balance is a problem a stationary seated bicycle is also helpful instead of a treadmill. The same place you find excellent treadmills will carry excellent recumbent stationary bikes.

FITT Definition

FITT is a government acronym for exercise indicating the Frequency, Intensity, Time (or duration) and Type of exercise. A number of studies have simplified this for us today.

Our FITT parameters can be defined as follows:

For your **Less Fit Patients**:

Frequency: Daily so 3-5-7 Days a week
Intensity   2-3 miles per hour on a treadmill or track
Time: 30-60 minutes Duration
Type: Walking

For your **More Fit Patients**:

Frequency: Daily so 7 Days a week
Intensity   4 miles per hour on a treadmill or track
Time: 1 Hour Duration
Type: Brisk Walking

For your patients who are **Very Fit but cannot get to that ideal weight:**

Frequency: Daily so 7 Days a week – TWICE a day
Intensity   4-5+ miles per hour on a treadmill or track
Time: 1 Hour Duration
Type: Brisk Walking

Of course Very Fit patients can also do 1 hour twice a day of cardio-kickboxing or step aerobics or spinning (stationary cycling).

How did we come to these numbers? From the most current research and information on what protects and what does not protect.
Now let's look at the appropriate studies:

1. Age-adjusted all-cause mortality rates declined across physical fitness quintiles from 64.0 per 10,000 person-years in the least fit men to 18.6 per 10,000 person-years in the most-fit men. Corresponding values for women were 39.5 per 10,000 person-years to 8.5 per 10,000 person-years[509]. That said, of everything we say in this book, of every point we make, THE MOST CRITICAL FACTOR that determines relative death rate and relative risk of various chronic diseases (CAD, diabetes, breast cancer, lung cancer, etc) even more so than cholesterol levels, blood sugars, hsCRP, and all other risk factors IS THE QUINTILE INTO WHICH YOUR PATIENTS FALL AS TO RELATIVE FITNESS LEVEL FOR THEIR AGE. After adjustment

for age, the peak exercise capacity measured in metabolic equivalents (MET) was the strongest predictor of the risk of death among both normal subjects and those with cardiovascular disease. Absolute peak exercise capacity was a stronger predictor of the risk of death than the percentage of the age-predicted value achieved, and there was no interaction between the use or nonuse of beta-blockade and the predictive power of exercise capacity. **Each 1-MET increase in exercise capacity conferred a 12 percent improvement in survival**[510]. If your patients are in the top quintile they have the lowest risk of death from every disease in the Top Ten list. We were not kidding when we said train your patients to be marathon runners or triathletes -- world class would be best. Short of this just getting them to 1-4-7 would be the minimum.

2. You should also know it is **current fitness level** not fitness level your patients were once at when they were in college[511] – this history seems to have no impact as we get older except though that as every athlete knows, muscles have memories and it is easier for pervious college athletes or patients who were athletes in their twenties to become fit again. So every athlete at a bar who likes to talk about their glory days they are just that – talkers with glory days with no impact on current health risks. Talk is cheap – working out is hard.

3. From Chapter One Prevention of a Cardiovascular Death we know the NEW Minimum for exercise frequency and duration came from the Institute of Medicine in 2002 which increased both to seven days a week for at least one hour each day (**1 hour a day 7 days a week**)[512]

4. We know from the Harvard Alumni Study that for every hour people exercise they live two hours[513] – that's **2 for 1**. It's a great payoff and one of the reasons the Institute of Medicine came out with their advice.

5. Compared with inactive individuals, those who walked at least 2 h/wk had a 39% lower all-cause mortality and a 34% lower CVD mortality rate. When controlled for sex, age, race, body mass index, smoking, and comorbid conditions. The mortality rates were lowest for persons who **walked 3 to 4 h/wk** and for those who reported that their walking involved moderate increases in heart and breathing rates[514].

6. Walking was associated with reduced risk of total stroke[515] (RRs across increasing walking MET quintiles, 1.00, 0. 76, 0.78, 0.70, and 0.66; P for trend=.01) and ischemic stroke (RRs across increasing walking MET quintiles, 1.00, 0.77, 0.75, 0.69, and 0.60; P for trend=.02). **Brisk or striding walking** pace was associated with lower risk of total and ischemic stroke compared with average or casual pace. Brisk walking has been long defined as >4 mph or >5.6 km/hr[516].

7. Both walking and vigorous exercise were associated with substantial reductions in the risk of coronary events. There was a strong, graded inverse relation between energy expenditure, either walking or vigorous exercise and the incidence of coronary events. Risk was reduced equally in women who **walked briskly** for at least 3 hours per week and women who exercised vigorously for 1.5 hours per week. As compared with women in the lowest quintile group for energy expenditure (expressed as the metabolic-equivalent [MET] score), women in increasing quintile groups had age-adjusted relative risks of 0.77, 0.65, 0.54, and 0.46 for coronary events (P for trend <0.001). In multivariate analyses, the inverse gradient remained strong (relative risks, 0.88, 0.81, 0.74, and 0.66 for women in increasing quintile groups as compared with those in the lowest quintile group; P for trend=0.002). Walking was inversely associated with the risk of coronary events; women in the highest quintile group for walking, who walked the equivalent of three or more hours per week at a brisk pace, had a multivariate relative risk of 0.65 as compared with women who walked infrequently. Regular vigorous exercise (≥6 MET) was associated with similar risk reductions (30 to 40 percent). Sedentary women who became active in middle adulthood or later had a lower risk of coronary events than their counterparts who remained sedentary[517].

8. A very large review of 10 prospective cohort studies of physical activity of moderate intensity and type 2 diabetes, including a total of 301,221 participants and 9,367 incident cases showed

adherence to recommendations to participate in physical activities of moderate intensity such as **brisk walking can substantially reduce the risk of type 2 diabetes**. The summary Relative Risk of type 2 diabetes was 0.69 for regular participation in physical activity of moderate intensity as compared with being sedentary[518].

9. Brisk walking can be an effective intervention for overweight/obese middle-aged women with hypertriglyceridemia in reducing cardiovascular risk by lowering triglyceride (TG) and Apo B levels. **Adding diet to brisk walking may have no additional significant effects on changes in TG and Apo B**[519].

Meshing all of this together we defined the FITT parameters which your patients, for the most part, need to become fit and lose weight: 1 hour a day, 4 mph, 7 days a week. This is as simple as we can make it.

Your patients can just walk on their treadmill but they need to kick it up just a hair every week. If they are young enough and able, they should do walking twice a day with some of it being a little faster each week and a little farther.

To reiterate -- ideally TO MAINTAIN WEIGHT AND NOT GAIN patients should be doing one hour sessions on a treadmill at 4 miles per hour every day with some light weight lifting BUT this may take a year or two to reach.

To reiterate -- ideally TO LOSE WEIGHT patients should be doing two separate one hour sessions on a treadmill at 4 miles per hour every day with some light weight lifting BUT this level of conditioning may take a year or two to reach.

Another Approach – Shape Up America -- Using a Pedometer and 10,000 Steps™

The Shape Up America® organization has also come up with a walking program called the 10,000 Step™ Program -- this is an anti-obesity initiative launched by former U.S. Surgeon General C. Everett Koop -- offering new evidence that overweight adults can learn coping skills to lose unwanted pounds and to keep the weight off indefinitely. The program utilizes a pedometer and involves always taking 10,000 steps per day. This Surgeon General's recommendation for physical activity is to add about 30 minutes of moderate intensity activity each day ON TOP of your patient's customary daily activities (which usually only takes one to about 900-3,000 steps a day at the most) but with the addition of 30 minutes of intense walking or treadmill use a day 10,000 steps can be reached.

A few points about this excellent program (borrowed from the Shape Up America! website[520]):

1. To burn the equivalent of walking 10,000 steps, your patient would have to exercise long enough to burn 500 calories.
2. It takes about six months to "lock in" a new behavior. Your patient should aim to do what is necessary to change their exercise behavior permanently. They should be prepared to dedicate themselves to their daily goal each day for a minimum of six months. If they do that, they are much more likely to maintain this goal permanently.
3. Walking 10,000 steps is the approximate equivalent of walking 5 miles. The distance covered depends on the length of your patient's stride. That is why it is approximate.
4. The pedometer should be clipped to their belt firmly and the belt buckled securely so it won't move around. The pedometer should be worn in a location above the hip so that it can detect the leg movement.
5. If your patient likes riding a stationary bike they need to realize exercising long enough to burn 100 calories is like walking 2000 steps. To burn the equivalent of walking 10,000 steps, they would have to exercise long enough to burn approximately 500 calories.

A Few Critical Points To Make – The 11 Step Program 120® Eating Plan

(We would like to thank Dr. Hugo Rodier for his sage advice and great article, "Practical Principles of Advising Patients in Nutrition[521]" from where most of these concepts were gathered together in an original and cohesive manner.)

1. It's your job as a primary care physician to convince your patients they are addicted to two white crystalline substances just about as deadly as some of the other white crystalline substances out there (i.e. cocaine and heroin) – refined sugar and refined flour. This may seem a little extreme but remind them that alcohol is nothing but fermented sugar that is also highly addictive as is sugar[522] – and ask them if they really truly want to save their lives because no one else can at this point, and if they really do then **they have to avoid sugars and white flours**.

2. Secondly, educate your patients about the fact that industries which process foods intentionally place even more addictive substances, like advanced glycosylated end-products, and high-fructose corn syrup, into these processed foods, increasing consumers' addictions[523] even more so and worsening their insulin receptor functionality and diabetes[524]. **Do not eat any processed foods – eat whole foods only!**

3. Third, point out that fats have been demonized by the popular media to the point that we totally avoid them now[525] and as a consequence we have been forced to turn to sugars. Fats are not bad – we actually need them – it's just the relatively new trans-fats[526] and saturated fats that are bad. Sugar is far worse. **So they must avoid sugars, trans-fats, and saturated fats.**

4. Fourth, explain how the fast food industry spends in excess of $33 billion dollars last year on advertising to capture your patient and their children[527] [528] into a quick and easy habit of eating incredibly unhealthy foods, an agenda based on profits not your patient's health, while the farmers of America only spend about $5 million a year to advertise fruits and vegetables. How about **when your patients need fast food instead they stop by the local market and grab some fruit and protein bars**?

5. Tell them to **quit supporting their local fast food establishments and soda-pop bottlers and distributors** and instead support their local fruit growers and produce stands. No more soda pops. **One apple-a-day instead** and they would have more money to eat better[529]!

6. **First Two –Eight Weeks**:
    - ❑ Along with STRICTLY following the Atkins Diet® your patients may also eat only vegetables, nuts, and lean meats (eggs are O.K.) They may eat avocados and tomatoes.
    - ❑ Salad dressing: olive oil, vinegar, pepper, lemons, tarragon, garlic.
    - ❑ Drinks: water with lemons, veggie juices (that they juice for themselves is best).
    - ❑ If an item is not on the list, it is to be avoided.

    (**Why this approach?** They are reducing their storages of glycogen, reducing insulin resistance peripherally, and centrally in the hypothalamus, and they are changing the way their taste buds perceive sugars, which must be done for their metabolisms to start changing. Their appetite thermostats are disrupted. They will never succeed, unless this is fixed[530].

    Plus, they are ridding themselves of their sugar addiction, which must be done aggressively, as with alcohol addictions.)

7. **Second Two Weeks**: Add all Fruits

8. **Third Two Weeks**: Add legumes, brown rice and whole grains.

9. **Forever:**
    - ❑ **No refined foods, soda pop, nor white flour (breads, pasta, candy, cakes, etc.)**
    - ❑ **Indiscretions: can they stop at one or two or will they relapse like an alcoholic?**

- ❑ **Stress management**: Many patients have personalities that cause their eating to be driven by stress. They must become aware of this, and deal with those issues more responsibly with hard exercise or meditation, etc.
- ❑ **Look in to HPA axis dysfunction**. Most abused children have a disruption of this axis, especially later as adults, which creates significant metabolic problems[531]. They must address these issues through counseling, or any other technique that will increase their sense of control, and forgiveness[532].
- ❑ **Never go hungry.** This will cause patients to eat what is convenient (fast food, refined food.) **Be proactive: carry nuts, veggies, and other convenient foods, such as Pulse® bars** (other bars are full of preservatives, and alcohol sugars).
- ❑ **Don't count calories. Restrictive diets don't work.** While counting calories may succeed in some people, this approach requires an iron will, which is rare in our society. Most people will have abandoned such diets within a year[533] [534]. Why would one stop eating when one is still hungry? Counting calories only makes sense when you have not fixed your fat thermostat. Addicted people cannot stop eating on their own. Their metabolic signals are so disturbed that their hunger is not slaked unless the addictive substances (e.g. refined sugars) are consumed. A vicious cycle is perpetuated. Counting calories is their only hope, unless they fix the thermostat, and rely on their "healthy hunger" to guide their choices[535].
- ❑ **Again, never go hungry: Filling up on the foods listed above (fruits, veggies, nuts, legumes, lean meats and whole grains)** without counting calories, will perpetuate their reliance on their hunger "to eat or not to eat." Have you ever seen anybody overdo those foods? "Welcome to the Mediterranean diet[536]."
- ❑ **Keep it simple: Leave the cooking up to your patients.**
- ❑ **Eat breakfast like a king, lunch like a queen, and dinner like a pauper.** Skipping breakfast causes more insulin resistance[537].
- ❑ **For best results, ask patients about their diets "at each visit."** "There is insufficient awareness on the part of physicians of the benefits of dietary treatment. Although dietitians do have an important role in patient care, the key to dietary changes is the repetition of dietary education by the Primary Care Provider at each visit[538]."
- ❑ **Never go hungry, don't count calories: the diet above is high in protein.** It has been shown to control hunger, and appetite a lot better:
- ❑ "A high protein diet induces sustained reductions in appetite ad libitum caloric intake, and body weight[539]."
- ❑ "Too restrictive?" Not really. **Patients are eager to hear from their doctors what to do to overcome chronic problems** *[the real point of this book – Program 120® Ed.]*. Dr. Hugo Rodier's experience[540] is full of examples of patients who are extremely thankful that someone has shown them the way out of significant suffering. He feels this simple approach works. Blood sugars are corrected, blood pressure falls up to 50 points, cholesterol problems go away, insulin resistance decreases, and practically all problems his patients face improve, particularly energy problems. All this is well outlined in the medical literature. After all, it all boils down to the "metabolomics[541]" of each person's cells.

10. Last -- this is all such a critical aspect of this entire lifestyle program that if they do not agree to these modifications, you will not take their case and they can go elsewhere for care.

11. Ask them about their eating during every time you see them. Give them a Program 120® Diet Log so you can see what they are doing and how much they are eating. This is a must. Night or sleep eaters[542] (also known as amnestic eaters) especially will not give you accurate logs, so beware.

Last Resort – Bariatric Surgery For The Desperate

Liposuction of the abdomen does not treat the real problem because the hormone resistin and the insulin resistance almost completely stems from omental fat. Many patients turn to bariatric surgery.

Bariatric Surgery – Overall Success

Modern bariatric surgery involves reducing the size of the gastric reservoir with or without associated malabsorption. These operations have lately achieved impressive results, with approximately a 50% or more reduction in excess body weight by 18-24 months post operation[543] but this is only true for up to 67 - 88% of the patients.

Indications

A body mass index (BMI) of 40 kg per m2 or greater, or 35 kg per m2 or greater with serious obesity-related comorbidities (e.g., diabetes, obstructive sleep apnea, coronary artery disease, debilitating arthritis) are baseline indications for the surgery[544] but not necessarily indications of successful weight loss or even survival after the surgery.

Indications for Bariatric Surgery from the National Institutes of Health[545]

1. BMI of 40 kg per m2 or higher, or BMI of 35 kg per m2 or higher with serious obesity-related comorbidities (e.g., diabetes, obstructive sleep apnea, coronary artery disease, debilitating arthritis)
2. Previous failed weight loss attempts involving an integrated nonsurgical weight loss program including dietary modification, behavioral support, and appropriate exercise
3. Possession of appropriate motivation and psychological stability to understand risks and benefits of the procedure as well as the commitment to lifelong postoperative lifestyle changes and medical surveillance

NOTE: A good candidate for bariatric surgery will meet *all three* indications.

Types of Surgery

There are multiple operative approaches, but two main principles exist in combination, or alone, in the various procedures: restriction and malabsorption[546]. The Roux-en-Y gastric bypass (RYGB) has become the most commonly performed procedure for patients undergoing bariatric surgery[547][548] because it has the advantages of providing a restrictive and a malabsorptive component to induce weight loss[549].

Restrictive Surgeries – VBG and adjustable gastric banding result in long-term weight loss of approximately 40 percent of excess body weight[550].

Malabsorptive Surgeries – RYGB and biliopancreatic diversion result in an average long-term weight loss of 60 percent[551].

Surgery for the Super Obese (BMI >50 kg/m2) -- biliopancreatic diversion, which is highly effective in super-obese patients (i.e., body mass index [BMI] higher than 50 kg per m2)[552].

Choosing The Right Patient For The Procedure

It is recommended that, before bariatric surgery, potential patients be evaluated by a team with medical, surgical, psychological, and nutritional expertise – careful motivational testing should be performed. Potential candidates for bariatric surgery should be selected carefully based on the NIH criteria (listed above) and only after a thorough multidisciplinary evaluation that especially determines if these patients will be likely to follow up properly[553] – this point cannot be stressed enough!

Hard Facts About Bariatric Surgery

Here's what the research shows:

1. According to the International Bariatric Surgery Registry, the leading cause of death following bariatric surgery is pulmonary embolism with risk factors including a BMI of 60 kg per m2 or higher (super obese patients), chronic lower extremity edema, obstructive sleep apnea, and previous pulmonary embolism[554]. Low-molecular-weight heparin and compression stockings should be used postoperatively to minimize risk of pulmonary embolism for most patients. Patients at moderate risk of pulmonary embolism should receive prophylactic doses of low-molecular-weight heparin (up to 3,400 U per day), whereas high-risk patients should be considered for therapeutic doses (more than 3,400 U per day)[555].

2. Anastomotic leaks and respiratory failure are other possible causes of death in patients who have had bariatric surgery -- signs of anastomotic leaks are sustained tachycardia, severe abdominal pain, fever, rigors, and hypotension[556].

3. Thirty-day mortality was 1.9% and was associated with surgical inexperience. Within the surgeon's first 19 procedures the odds of death within 30 days were 4.7 times higher than at later points in a surgeon's case order. At 15 years followup, 16.3% of nonoperated patients had died as compared with 11.8% of patients who had the bariatric procedure. Thirty-day mortality after gastric bypass is higher than previously reported and closely linked to surgeon inexperience. A modest overall survival benefit was associated with the procedure but a marked survival advantage was noted for patients who survive to the first postoperative year[557].

4. Some common short-term complications of bariatric surgery are wound infections, stomal stenosis (i.e., narrowing of the gastrojejunostomy), marginal ulceration, and constipation[558]. Wound infections are more common in open[559] than in laparoscopic procedures and may occur in up to 20 percent of patients[560].

5. What happens if you don't follow up after your bariatric surgery? Percentage excess body weight loss was greater in group that followed up as ordered plus more of these patients had successful weight loss (defined as within 50% of ideal body weight [88%] vs. 28 [67%]). This study[561] found that a significant number of patients will not comply with regular follow-up care after laparoscopic gastric bypass unless they are prompted to do so by their bariatric clinic. These patients have worse clinical outcome (i.e., less weight loss). Caution should be taken when examining the results of any bariatric study where there is a significant loss to follow-up.

6. Look at the above numbers again – only 88% of those who did follow-up got to within 50% of their ideal body weight[562]. Only 88%? And "within 50% of their ideal body weight"? And only 67% of the others? So if your ideal body weight is 180 lbs does that mean only 67-88% got to within 50% of that number (270 lbs?)? That does not seem to be very good for the 4+% death risk (in the first 30 days) most patients take. Clearly you must tell your patients that it is not 100% effective with all patients.

7. Constipation is a common short-term consequence of bariatric surgery. Stemming from this there lately have been a number of reports of bowel obstructions in patients with RYGB[563] some cases even leading to intussusception.

8. Complications which can occur in the long term are symptomatic cholelithiasis, dumping syndrome, persistent vomiting, and nutritional deficiencies.

   ❑ Cholelithiasis is a common consequence of rapid weight loss in the postoperative period and occurs in up to 50 percent of patients[564]. Prophylactic cholecystectomy during the surgery or the use of bile salt therapy remain the mainstays of treatment.

   ❑ Dumping syndrome is a constellation of procholinergic symptoms resulting from an influx of undigested carbohydrates into the jejunum and is usually a side effect of malabsorptive bariatric procedures such as RYGB and biliopancreatic diversion. Symptoms include nausea, vomiting, diarrhea, tachycardia, salivation, and dizziness. It results from poor dietary compliance and can serve as a motivational tool for patients to avoid nonpermissible foods[565]. It is self-limited and usually subsides one to two hours after consuming sweet foods or those high in simple carbohydrates[566].

9. Pouch distension is another complication. It is critical that these patients adhere to specific dietary recommendations knowing that failure to do so may result in episodes of vomiting caused by pouch distention[567]. These patients require lifelong adjustment in eating behavior, including cutting food into small portions, chewing food thoroughly before swallowing, eating slowly, and waiting one hour after a meal before drinking anything – if they are not willing to comply with these behaviors then do not refer them for this surgery.

10. Protein-calorie malnutrition can occur in a few patients months to years after surgery because of anastomotic strictures or food phobias. Typically, these patients have had repeated episodes of nausea and daily vomiting and multiple hospitalizations for dehydration, renal insufficiency, and liver failure. Remember, the first and most important step is to reverse the protein-calorie malnutrition by aggressive total parenteral nutrition, dilation of strictures, and later institution of enteral nutrition until all the physical and biochemical manifestations of malnutrition have resolved[568]. Do not make the inexperienced mistake of first reflexively reversing the procedure.

11. For follow up to be truly effective it must involve a consistent multidisciplinary approach. The program you choose should be heavily researched for complication rates (mortality and morbidity) and the aggressiveness of the long term (two to three years minimum) follow-up with a team consisting of a bariatrician, dieticians, nutritionists, endocrinologists and psychological counseling as advised by the Mayo Clinic[569] and the American Society of Bariatric Physicians.

Common Monitoring Parameters for Bariatric Surgery Patients[570]

Every three months for first year -- Complete blood count, glucose, creatinine

Every six months for first year -- Liver function tests, protein and albumin, iron, total iron-binding capacity, ferritin, vitamin B12, folic acid, calcium, parathyroid hormone (if hypercalcemic).

Every year after the first year -- All of the above laboratory tests

Conclusion on Bariatric Surgery

Though the perioperative mortality of bariatric surgery *in the hands of a skilled experienced surgeon* is less than 1%[571] but this can be much higher when a surgeon has done less than 100 bariatric procedures – in this situation up to 4.4% of patients can die in the first 30 days! It is the conclusion of the Program 120® team that bariatric surgery works for the majority of patients those who are morbidly obese but, in light of all of the really horrendous late complications that are not clearly addressed in the literature and the severity of the surgery and subsequent common complications and morbidity, this should be considered as a last resort.

If your patient wants surgery regardless here's what you tell them before you agree to the referral:

Four Rules For Patient Success With Bariatric Surgery

1. Experience counts and can lessen your death risk by 75%! You must choose an experienced bariatric surgeon and team who's been involved with hundreds of cases not just a few (>100).

2. What's the 30 day mortality rate of the program you picked? It should be less than 1%. If the hospital and team won't tell you in writing then do not go there.

3. Part of this selection process is evaluating in advance their multidisciplinary team who performs the follow-up – who are they and what kind of experience do they have? Is there a member of the American Society of Bariatric Physicians in the group? What kind of vitamin deficiencies do they regularly look for? What kind of follow up do they require?

4. You must follow up with the multidisciplinary team for all visits after your surgery! This means success if you go, or failure or even death if you don't!

The Program 120® Lifestyle That Really Works

Considering all the research we've quoted and noted here's an easy to follow plan that works but is not too Spartan for most.

1. Order a ECG-Gated 64-MDCT scan (64 slice CAT scan) or cIMT (see Chapter 1 Cardiovascular Disease for details) to rule out heart disease. Skip this if your patient has no cardiac risk factors. This way both you, as their physician, and your hard working patient know they are not going to keel over in the middle of a 4 mile 1 hour brisk walk you prescribed.

2. Make sure they know this is going to be hard work and can take years to reshape the body they abused for so long. If they're not committed do not bother pursuing this regimen.

3. Start on the proper preventive meds and nutraceuticals as detailed in the appropriate chapters of this book looking especially the CVD risk precautions.

4. Your patients should also be on proper modern HRT – this is to your patient's advantage and can vastly improve their insulin receptor functionality and ability to exercise and to recover more quickly from arduous exercise.

5. Start them on The 10 Step Program 120® Eating Plan as detailed above. Ask about this every time you see them. Follow their diet logs.

6. Start them on The Program 120® 1-4-7 FITT Plan for exercise – give them a written prescription detailing what they are supposed to do and how often.

The rest will be automatic.

PROGRAM 120® CHECKLIST

☐ Get a **ECG-Gated 64-MDCT scan** (64 slice CAT scan) or cIMT as ordered by your physician to rule out heart disease. *[+15-20]*

☐ Carbohydrates are absolutely poison for most humans – consider them to be and you will be much healthier. *[+20-30 (yrs) or more!]*

☐ Your physician has written you an exercise prescription for an exercise program such as -- **The Program 120® 1-4-7 FITT Plan** -- do it – never stop! *[+15-20]*

☐ You have been prescribed **The 11 Step Program 120® Eating Plan** to follow – do it – you will not be hungry. *[+15-20]*

☐ Overall modify your lifestyle – SAVE YOUR LIFE—you now have **The Program 120® Lifestyle Plan** – it works – use it. *[+15-20]*

☐ Get your hormone levels checked and make sure you're levels are optimized – especially thyroid and IGF-1. *[+15-20]*

☐ Though considered food supplements get on DHEA and melatonin at the doses your doctor trained in anti-aging and wellness medicine approves. *[+5-10]*

☐ Drink purified or bottled water only. Keep some always in your house and car. *[+5-10]*

- [ ] Every one needs good bowel flora – take a probiotic like Natren's Healrhy Trinity™ at least once a week – more often if you have taken antibiotics.. *[+2-10]*
- [ ] Eat at least 8-15 raw blanched almonds every day. *[+2-5]*
- [ ] Take high quality fish oil 1000 mgm or more every day (usually at least two capsules per day of the higher quality supplements). *[+5-10]*
- [ ] Add almonds and berries and whole grains to your diet. *[+15-20]*
- [ ] Buy a quality treadmill for use every day. *[+10-20]*
- [ ] If you have Metabolic Syndrome lose weight NOW – go to a diet boot camp, cut your calories in half – do something!!!! *[+25-30]*
- [ ] Really obese and nothing else works? Try bariatric surgery but beware of the risks. Makes sure you get long and appropriate follow-up by someone who's qualified. *[+5-10]*

Top Ten Program 120® Preventive Steps

1. If you smoke QUIT! If you smoke occasionally and at a bar or parties QUIT that too.

2. If you've never smoked avoid secondhand smoke. Remember exercising can increase your chance of quitting by up to 80 %!

3. Exercise at least 1 hour a day—with a goal of walking/jogging at least 4 mph on a treadmill. Light weights for three times a week at least.

4. Eat right! Mediterranean, Caveman or Zone® lifestyle diets preferred! Lots of olive oil, olives, almonds (blanched or raw), and fresh fruit and vegetables!

5. Take the right kind of vitamins: A No copper, No iron vitamin is ideal

    i. Calcium-Magnesium (not carbonate) twice a day
    ii. Vitamins D3 and K2
    iii. Extra Vitamin E and C
    iv. High quality molecularly distilled fish oil capsule (2,500 mg DHA+EPA) a day.

6. Add rosuvastatin (Crestor®), even if it's a tiny dose, to your regimen—this cools the endothelium, prevents stroke and heart disease, and reduces cancer risk. (Simvastatin is another option)

7. Add Niaspan® to your regimen! Forget the flushing – this high dose niacin lowers the bad HDL (apo B) and LDL cholesterol and lowers triglycerides while elevating the good HDL! This stuff has been around for decades but still rocks!

8. Optimize your hormones using biologically identical human hormones (as we've detailed in this book) – you will feel better (improves quality of life), be able to exercise longer and more effectively, reduce multiple risk factors, and have better skin, better arteries, better bones, better brain function/cognition, and better balance, and be generally much healthier.

9. Filter your drinking water and air in your car and home – keep a watch on these basic things – they make a huge difference.

10. If you have high blood pressure get it under perfect control – 120/70. To do this you should use an ARB such as the telmisartan (Micardis®) or telmisartan plus HCTZ (hydrochlorothiazide or Micardis-HCT®). And don't forget that an appropriate dose of melatonin taken at night can help bring your blood pressure down.

Bonus EXTRA: We don't really discuss this in the book but are big believers in this for your health-- avoid bad decisions that lead to moral and personal struggles – these cause you stress and misery which can really damage your body through a number of pathways. Hearken back to your family values inculcated at youth – that's where you should be. If you weren't raised to make wise personal decisions (like don't have that unprotected sex! And don't drink that vodka! Don't do those drugs!) then change now. You'll be healthier and happier. Watch for our upcoming Program 120® Guide for Youth! Watch for our upcoming Program 120® Guide for the Soul!

We love you all and wish you success in your attempts to get healthier and happier!

The Program 120® Team

A note from Dr. Purser

If you enjoyed this book and found it helpful please feel free to leave a review on Amazon on my Kindle book page (under the book title). It is MUCH appreciated and puts you in the running to win other free books with contests we occasionally have (in the future).

If you wish to order this book in paperback please go to my website and order it there:

www.danpursermd.com

Also, if your physician won't or can't (as is often the case nowadays) order you the specific labs you request (which I suggest in this book) – on the above website you will also see a button for Direct Labs – just click on that and follow their directions. It is a cheap and easy way to get labs locally near you and to pay cash (actually a credit card I believe) – just know that insurance will not cover these nor can you get reimbursed as no diagnostic code will be issued (how can we? We don't even know you nor have we seen you…).

☺

Thanks so much for purchasing AND reading this book – your seeking for knowledge in a confusing world is much appreciated.

--Dan Purser, MD

PS Like me on Facebook too – I try to answer all questions I get there (if I can legally).

[1] Beck-Peccoz P, Mannavola D, Persani L. Syndromes of thyroid hormone resistance. Ann Endocrinol (Paris). 2005 Jun;66(3):264-9.

[2] Hulley S, Grady D, Bush T, et al. Randomized trial of estrogen plus progestin for secondary prevention of coronary heart disease in postmenopausal women: Heart and Estrogen/progestin Replacement Study (HERS) Research Group. JAMA 1998;280:605-613.

[3] [no author listed] Findings from the WHI Postmenopausal Hormone Therapy Trials. Available online at www.nhlbi.nih.gov/whi/. Accessed 2006 Sep 10.

[4] Meieran SE; Reus VI; Webster R; Shafton R; Wolkowitz OM. Chronic pregnenolone effects in normal humans: attenuation of benzodiazepine-induced sedation. Psychoneuroendocrinology. 2004; 29(4):486-500 (ISSN: 0306-4530).

[5] Morley JE, et al. Potentially predictive and manipulable blood serum correlates of aging in the healthy human male: Progressive decreases in bioavailable testosterone, dehydroepiandrosterone sulfate, and the ratio of insulin-like growth factor 1 to growth hormone. PNAS 1997;94;7537-7542.

[6] Veiga S ; Garcia-Segura LM ; Azcoitia I. Neuroprotection by the steroids pregnenolone and dehydroepiandrosterone is mediated by the enzyme aromatase. J Neurobiol. 2003; 56(4):398-406 (ISSN: 0022-3034).

[7] Flood JF ; Morley JE ; Roberts E. Pregnenolone sulfate enhances post-training memory processes when injected in very low doses into limbic system structures: the amygdala is by far the most sensitive. Proc Natl Acad Sci U S A. 1995; 92(23):10806-10 (ISSN: 0027-8424).

[8] Guth L ; Zhang Z ; Roberts E. Key role for pregnenolone in combination therapy that promotes recovery after spinal cord injury. Proc Natl Acad Sci U S A. 1994; 91(25):12308-12 (ISSN: 0027-8424).

[9] Tennant F, et al. Physiologic abnormalities as biologic markers in severe intractable pain. Program and abstracts of the 25th Annual Meeting of the American Pain Society; March 20-23, 2003; Chicago, Illinois.

[10] Darnaudéry M ; Koehl M ; Piazza PV ; Le Moal M ; Mayo W. Pregnenolone sulfate increases hippocampal acetylcholine release and spatial recognition. Brain Res. 2000; 852(1):173-9 (ISSN: 0006-8993).

[11] Schaeffer V, Patte-Mensah C, Eckert A, Mensah-Nyagan AG. Modulation of neurosteroid production in human neuroblastoma cells by Alzheimer's disease key proteins. J Neurobiol. 2006 Jul;66(8):868-81.

[12] Malhotra, S; Sawhney, G; Pandhi, P. MedGenMed Neurology & Neurosurgery -- The Therapeutic Potential of Melatonin: A Review of the Science. Medscape General Medicine. 2004;6(2):46. ©2004 Medscape Posted 04/13/2004. Available online at www.medscape.com/viewarticle/472385.

[13] Arendt J. Melatonin. Clin Endocrinol. 1998;29:205-229.

[14] Stetinova V, Smetanova L, Grossmann V, Anzenbacher P. In vitro and in vivo assessment of the antioxidant activity of melatonin and related indole derivatives. Gen Physiol Biophys. 2002;21:153-162.

[15] Reiter RJ, Tan DX, Leon J, Kilic U, Kilic E. When melatonin gets on your nerves: its beneficial actions in experimental models of stroke. Exp Biol Med (Maywood). 2005 Feb;230(2):104-17.

[16] Mayo JC, Sainz RM, Antolin I, Herrera F, Martin V, Rodriguez C. Melatonin regulation of antioxidant enzyme gene expression. Cell Mol Life Sci. 2002;59:1706-1713.

[17] Vogler B, Rapoport AM, Tepper SJ, Sheftell F, Bigal ME. Role of melatonin in the pathophysiology of migraine: implications for treatment. CNS Drugs. 2006;20(5):343-50.

[18] Peres MF, Masruha MR, Zukerman E, Moreira-Filho CA, Cavalheiro EA. Potential therapeutic use of melatonin in migraine and other headache disorders. Expert Opin Investig Drugs. 2006 Apr;15(4):367-75.

[19] Lissoni P, Chilelli M, Villa S, Cerizza L, Tancini G. Five years survival in metastatic non-small cell lung cancer patients treated with chemotherapy alone or chemotherapy and melatonin: a randomized trial. J Pineal Res. 2003 Aug;35(1):12-5.

[20] Nishida S. Metabolic effects of melatonin on oxidative stress and diabetes mellitus. Endocrine. 2005 Jul;27(2):131-6.

[21] Head KA. Natural therapies for ocular disorders, part two: cataracts and glaucoma. Altern Med Rev. 2001 Apr;6(2):141-66.

[22] Pandi-Perumal SR, Srinivasan V, Maestroni GJ, Cardinali DP, Poeggeler B, Hardeland R. Melatonin. FEBS J. 2006 Jul;273(13):2813-38.

[23] Nishida S. Metabolic effects of melatonin on oxidative stress and diabetes mellitus. Endocrine. 2005 Jul;27(2):131-6.

[24] Ahmed HH, Mannaa F, Elmegeed GA, Doss SH. Cardioprotective activity of melatonin and its novel

synthesized derivatives on doxorubicin-induced cardiotoxicity. Bioorg Med Chem. 2005 Mar 1;13(5):1847-57.

[25] Brusco LI, Marquez M, Cardinali DP. Melatonin treatment stabilizes chronobiologic and cognitive symptoms in Alzheimer's disease. Neuroendocrinol Lett. 2000;21:39-423.

[26] Srinivasan V, Pandi-Perumal S, Cardinali D, Poeggeler B, Hardeland R. Melatonin in Alzheimer's disease and other neurodegenerative disorders. Behav Brain Funct. 2006 May 4;2(1):15.

[27] Bellon A. Searching for new options for treating insomnia: are melatonin and ramelteon beneficial? J Psychiatr Pract. 2006 Jul;12(4):229-43.

[28] Lewy AJ, Emens J, Jackman A, Yuhas K. Circadian uses of melatonin in humans. Chronobiol Int. 2006;23(1-2):403-12.

[29] Bellon A. Searching for new options for treating insomnia: are melatonin and ramelteon beneficial? J Psychiatr Pract. 2006 Jul;12(4):229-43.

[30] Kunz D, Mahlberg R, Muller C, Tilmann A, Bes F. Melatonin in patients with reduced REM sleep duration: two randomized controlled trials. J Clin Endocrinol Metab. 2004 Jan;89(1):128-34.

[31] Bella LD, Gualano L. Key Aspects of Melatonin Physiology: Thirty Years of Research. Neuro Endocrinol Lett. 2006 Aug 5;27(4).

[32] Bartsch C, Bartsch H. The anti-tumor activity of pineal melatonin and cancer enhancing life styles in industrialized societies. Cancer Causes Control. 2006 May;17(4):559-71.

[33] Rimler A, Lupowitz Z, Zisapel N. Differential regulation by melatonin of cell growth and androgen receptor binding to the androgen response element in prostate cancer cells. Neuroendocrinol Lett. 2002;23(suppl 1):45-49.

[34] Sainz RM, Mayo JC, Tan DX, Leon J, Manchester L, Reiter RJ. Melatonin reduces prostate cancer cell growth leading to neuroendocrine differentiation via a receptor and PKA independent mechanism. Prostate. 2005 Apr 1;63(1):29-43.

[35] Karasek M, Carillo-Vico A, Guerrero JM, Winczyk K, Pawlikowsky M. Expression of melatonin MT(1) and MT(2) receptors, and ROR alpha(1) receptor in transplantable murine Colon 38 cancer. Neuroendocrinol Lett. 2002;23(suppl 1):55-60.

[36] Wenzel U, Nickel A, Daniel H. Melatonin potentiates flavone-induced apoptosis in human colon cancer cells by increasing the level of glycolytic end products. Int J Cancer. 2005 Aug 20;116(2):236-42. Copyright 2005 Wiley-Liss, Inc

[37] Scheer FA; Van Montfrans GA; van Someren EJ; Mairuhu G; Buijs RM. Daily nighttime melatonin reduces blood pressure in male patients with essential hypertension. Hypertension. 2004; 43(2):192-7 (ISSN: 1524-4563).

[38] Drake MJ, Mills IW, Noble JG. Melatonin pharmacotherapy for nocturia in men with benign prostatic enlargement. J Urol. 2004 Mar;171(3):1199-202.

[39] Nava M, Quirozz Y, Vaziri ND, Rodriguez-Iturbe B. Melatonin reduces renal interstitial inflammation and improves hypertension in spontaneously hypertensive rats. Am J Physiol Renal Physiol. 2002.

[40] Mayo JC, Sainz RM, Antolin I, Herrera F, Martin V, Rodriguez C. Melatonin regulation of antioxidant enzyme gene expression. Cell Mol Life Sci. 2002;59:1706-1713.

[41] Chen Q, Wei W. Effects and mechanisms of melatonin on inflammatory and immune responses of adjuvant arthritis rat. Int Immunopharmacol. 2002;2:1443-1449.

[42] Mayo JC, Sainz RM, Antolin I, Herrera F, Martin V, Rodriguez C. Melatonin regulation of antioxidant enzyme gene expression. Cell Mol Life Sci. 2002;59:1706-1713.

[43] Chen Q, Wei W. Effects and mechanisms of melatonin on inflammatory and immune responses of adjuvant arthritis rat. Int Immunopharmacol. 2002;2:1443-1449.

[44] Scheer FA; Van Montfrans GA; van Someren EJ; Mairuhu G; Buijs RM. Daily nighttime melatonin reduces blood pressure in male patients with essential hypertension. Hypertension. 2004; 43(2):192-7 (ISSN: 1524-4563).

[45] Cagnacci A, Cannoletta M, Renzi A, Baldassari F, Arangino S, Volpe A. Prolonged melatonin administration decreases nocturnal blood pressure in women. Am J Hypertens. 2005 Dec;18(12 Pt 1):1614-8.

[46] Todisco M, Casaccia P, Rossi N. Severe bleeding symptoms in refractory idiopathic thrombocytopenic purpura: a case successfully treated with melatonin. Am J Ther. 2003 Mar-Apr;10(2):135-6.

[47] Mahmoud F, Sarhill N, Mazurczak MA. The therapeutic application of melatonin in supportive care and palliative medicine. J Hosp Palliat Care. 2005 Jul-Aug;22(4):295-309.

[48] [No authors listed] Ramelteon (Rozerem) for insomnia. Med Lett Drugs Ther. 2005 Nov 7;47(1221):89-91.

[49] Lewy AJ, Sack RL. Phase typing and bright light therapy of chronobiologic sleep and mood disorders. In: Angelos, H, ed. Chronobiology and Psychiatric Disorders. New York, NY: Elsevier; 1987:181-206.

[50] The Journal of Immunology. Copyright © 2003 by The American Association of Immunologists, Inc. The Journal of Immunology, 2003, 171: 5157–5164.

[51] Walker, BD. Immune Reconstitution and Immunotherapy in HIV Infection. [online] Available on Medscape at www.medscape.com/viewprogram/2435. Accessed 2006 Sep 8.

[52] Gutierrez, MA; Stimmel, GL. Management of and Counseling for Psychotropic Drug-Induced Sexual Dysfunction. Pharmacotherapy 19(7):823-831, 1999. © 1999 Pharmacotherapy Publications.

[53] Baulieu EE. Dehydroepiandrosterone (DHEA): a fountain of youth? J Clin Endocrinol Metab 1996;81:3147-51.

[54] Regelson W, Loria R, Kalimi M. Hormonal intervention: "buffer hormones" or "state dependency." The role of dehydro-epiandrosterone (DHEA), thyroid hormone, estrogen and hypophysectomy in aging. Ann NY Acad Sci 1988;521:260-73.

[55] Cameron DR, Braunstein GD. The use of dehydroepiandrosterone therapy in clinical practice. Treat Endocrinol. 2005;4(2):95-114.

[56] Cameron DR, Braunstein GD. The use of dehydroepiandrosterone therapy in clinical practice. Treat Endocrinol. 2005;4(2):95-114.

[57] Brown GA, Vukovich M, King DS. Testosterone prohormone supplements. Med Sci Sports Exerc. 2006 Aug;38(8):1451-61

[58] Zdrojewicz Z ; Kesik S.[Dehydroepiandrosterone (DHEA)--youth hormone?] Wiad Lek. 2001; 54(11-12):693-704 (ISSN: 0043-5147). Available online at www.medsape.com. Accessed 2006 Sep 4.

[59] Morales AJ, Haubrich RH, Hwang JY, Asakura H, Yen SS. The Effect of Six Months Treatment With a 100 mg Daily Dose of Dehydroepiandrosterone (DHEA) on Circulating Sex Steroids, Body Composition and Muscle Strength in Age-Advanced Men and Women. Clin Endocrinol (Oxf). 1998;49(4):421-432.

[60] Furutama D, Fukui R, Amakawa M, Ohsawa N. Inhibition of migration and proliferation of vascular smooth muscle cells by dehydroepiandrosterone sulfate. Biochim Biophys Acta. 1998 Feb 27;1406(1):107-14.

[61] Herrington DM. Dehydroepiandrosterone and coronary atherosclerosis. Ann N Y Acad Sci. 1995 Dec 29;774:271-80.

[62] Barret-Connor E, Knaw KT, Yen SSC. A prospective study of dehydroepiandrosterone sulfate, mortality and cardiovascular disease. N Engl J Med. 1986 Dec 11; 315:1519-24.

[63] Nestler JE. Regulation of human dehydroepiandrosterone metabolism by insulin. Ann NY Acad Sci 1995;774:73-81.

[64] Villareal DT, Holloszy JO. Effect of DHEA on abdominal fat and insulin action in elderly women and men: a randomized controlled trial. JAMA. 2004 Nov 10;292(18):2243-8.

[65] Derksen RH. Dehydroepiandrosterone (DHEA) and systemic lupus erythematosus. Semin Arthritis Rheum. 1998; 27:335-47.

[66] Rabkin JG, Ferrando SJ, Wagner GJ et al. DHEA treatment for HIV+ patients: effects on mood, androgenic and anabolic parameters. Psychoneuroendocrinology. 2000; 25(1):53-68.

[67] Vermeulen A, Kaufman JM, Giagulli VA. Influence of some biological indexes on sex hormone-binding globulin and androgen levels in aging or obese males. J Clin Endocrinol Metab. 1996;81:1821-1826.

[68] Villareal DT. Effects of dehydroepiandrosterone on bone mineral density: what implications for therapy? Treat Endocrinol. 2002;1(6):349-57.

[69] Perrini S ; Laviola L ; Natalicchio A ; Giorgino F. Associated hormonal declines in aging: DHEAS. J Endocrinol Invest. 2005; 28(3 Suppl):85-93 (ISSN: 0391-4097).

[70] Arlt W. Dehydroepiandrosterone replacement therapy. Semin Reprod Med. 2004 Nov;22(4):379-88.

[71] Eser D, Schule C, Baghai TC, Romeo E, Uzunov DP, Rupprecht R. Neuroactive steroids and affective disorders. Pharmacol Biochem Behav. 2006 Jul 8.

[72] Wolkowitz OM, Reus VI, Roberts E, Manfredi F, Chan T, Raum WJ, Ormiston S, Johnson R, Canick J, Brizendine L, Weingartner H. Dehydroepiandrosterone (DHEA) treatment of depression. Biol Psychiatry. 1997 Feb 1;41(3):311-8.

[73] Barrett-Connor, E. (1992) Lower endogenous androgen levels and dyslipidemia in men with non insulin-

dependent diabetes mellitus. Annals of Internal Medicine, 117, 807–811.

[74] Villareal DT, Holloszy JO. Effect of DHEA on abdominal fat and insulin action in elderly women and men: a randomized controlled trial. JAMA. 2004 Nov 10;292(18):2243-8.

[75] Hirshman E; Wells E; Wierman ME; Anderson B; Butler A; Senholzi M; Fisher J. The effect of dehydroepiandrosterone (DHEA) on recognition memory decision processes and discrimination in postmenopausal women.
Psychon Bull Rev. 2003; 10(1):125-34 (ISSN: 1069-9384).

[76] Brooke AM, Kalingag LA, Miraki-Moud F, Camacho-Hubner C, Maher KT, Walker DM, Hinson JP, Monson JP. Dehydroepiandrosterone (DHEA) improves psychological well-being in male and female hypopituitary patients on maintenance growth hormone replacement. J Clin Endocrinol Metab. 2006 Jul 18.

[77] Williams JR. The effects of dehydroepiandrosterone on carcinogenesis, obesity, the immune system, and aging. Lipids. 2000 Mar;35(3):325-31.

[78] Lahita RG. Dehydroepiandrosterone (DHEA) for serious disease, a possibility? Lupus. 1999; 8:169-70.

[79] Villareal DT. Effects of dehydroepiandrosterone on bone mineral density: what implications for therapy? Treat Endocrinol. 2002;1(6):349-57.

[80] Morales AJ, Haubrich RH, Hwang JY, Asakura H, Yen SS. The Effect of Six Months Treatment With a 100 mg Daily Dose of Dehydroepiandrosterone (DHEA) on Circulating Sex Steroids, Body Composition and Muscle Strength in Age-Advanced Men and Women. Clin Endocrinol (Oxf). 1998;49(4):421-432.

[81] Williams CL, Stancel GM. Estrogens and progestins. In: Hardman JG, Limbird LE, Molinoff PB, Rudden RW, eds. Goodman and Gilman's the Pharmacological Basis for Therapeutics. New York, NY: McGraw-Hill; 1996:1411-1440.

[82] Finckh A, Berner IC, Aubry-Rozier B, So AK. A randomized controlled trial of dehydroepiandrosterone in postmenopausal women with fibromyalgia. J Rheumatol. 2005 Jul;32(7):1336-40.

[83] Stanczyk FZ. Best Pract Res Clin Endocrinol Metab. 2006 Jun;20(2):177-91. Diagnosis of hyperandrogenism: biochemical criteria.

[84] Bauer ME. Stress, glucocorticoids and ageing of the immune system. Stress. 2005; 8(1):69-83 (ISSN: 1025-3890).

[85] van Niekerk JK; Huppert FA; Herbert J. Salivary cortisol and DHEA: association with measures of cognition and well-being in normal older men, and effects of three months of DHEA supplementation. Psychoneuroendocrinology. 2001; 26(6):591-612 (ISSN: 0306-4530).

[86] Barclay, L. Medscape Medical News. Prasterone Helpful in Systemic Lupus Erythematosus. [online] Available at www.medscape.com/viewarticle/488995. Accessed 2006 Sep 4.

[87] Lobo, R. Menopause Management for the Millennium. [online] Available at www.medscape.com/viewprogram/213_pnt. Accessed 2006 Sep 4.

[88] Labrie F. Dehydroepiandrosterone, androgens and the mammary gland. Gynecol Endocrinol. 2006 Mar;22(3):118-30.

[89] Kehinde EO, Akanji AO, Al-Hunayan A, Memon A, Luqmani Y, Al-Awadi KA, Varghese R, Bashir AA, Daar AS. Do differences in age specific androgenic steroid hormone levels account for differing prostate cancer rates between Arabs and Caucasians? Int J Urol. 2006 Apr;13(4):354-61.

[90] Bunevicius R, Kazanavicius G, Zalinkevicius R, Prange AJ Jr. Effects of thyroxine as compared with thyroxine plus triiodothyronine in patients with hypothyroidism. N Engl J Med. 1999 Feb 11;340(6):424-9.

[91] Escobar-Morreale, H. F., Botella-Carretero, J. I., del Rey, F. E., de Escobar, G. M. (2005). Treatment of Hypothyroidism with Combinations of Levothyroxine plus Liothyronine. *J Clin Endocrinol Metab* 90: 4946-4954

[92] Escobar-Morreale, H. F., Botella-Carretero, J. I., Gomez-Bueno, M., Galan, J. M., Barrios, V., Sancho, J. (2005). Thyroid Hormone Replacement Therapy in Primary Hypothyroidism: A Randomized Trial Comparing L-Thyroxine plus Liothyronine with L-Thyroxine Alone. *Ann Intern Med* 142: 412-424

[93] Hennemann, G. Thyroxine Plus Low-Dose, Slow-Release Triiodothyronine Replacement in Hypothyroidism: Proof of Principle. Thyroid. Apr 2004, Vol. 14, No. 4: 271 -275.

[94] www.synthroidclaims.com

[95] Beckett GJ, Toft AD First-line thyroid function tests-TSH alone is not enough
Clin Endocrinol 2003; 56; 20-1.

[96] Arafah B. M. Increased Need for Thyroxine in Women with Hypothyroidism during Estrogen Therapy. N Engl J Med 2001; 344:1743-1749, Jun 7, 2001.

[97] AHFS Drug Information.(68:36.04 Thyroid Agents.) AHFS Drug Information (2004). Via Stat!Ref online. Available at: http://online.statref.com/. Accessed on November 23, 2004.

[98] [no author listed] What is Subclinical Hypothyroidism? Medical Crossfire. December 2000; Vol 2, No 12.

[99] Walsh, JP; Bremner,AP; Bulsara, MK; O'Leary, P; Leedman, PJ; Feddema, P; Michelangeli, V. Thyroid Dysfunction and Serum Lipids: A Community-Based Study. Clin Endocrinol. 2005;63(3):670-675. ©2005 Blackwell Publishing.

[100] Walsh, JP; Bremner,AP; Bulsara, MK; O'Leary, P; Leedman, PJ; Feddema, P; Michelangeli, V. Thyroid Dysfunction and Serum Lipids: A Community-Based Study. Clin Endocrinol. 2005;63(3):670-675. ©2005 Blackwell Publishing.

[101] Cappola, A.R. & Ladenson, P.W. (2003) Hypothyroidism and atherosclerosis. Journal of Clinical Endocrinology and Metabolism, 88, 2438– 2444.

[102] Cappola, A.R. & Ladenson, P.W. (2003) Hypothyroidism and atherosclerosis. Journal of Clinical Endocrinology and Metabolism, 88, 2438– 2444.

[103] Landenson PW. Recognition and management of cardiovascular disease related to thyroid dysfunction. Am J Med 1990;88:638-41.

[104] Hamilton MA, Stevenson LW, Fonarow GC, Steimle A, Goldhaber JI, Child JS, Chopra IJ, Moriguchi JD, Hage A. Safety and hemodynamic effects of intravenous triiodothyronine in advanced congestive heart failure. Am J Cardiol. 1998 Feb 15;81(4):443-7.

[105] P. Saravanan, W.-F. Chau, N. Roberts, K. Vedhara, R. Greenwood and C. M. Dayan. (2002) Psychological well-being in patients on 'adequate' doses of l-thyroxine: results of a large, controlled community-based questionnaire study. *Clinical Endocrinology* 57:5, 577-585

[106] Cooper, DS. Subclinical Thyroid Disease: A Clinician's Perspective. Annals of Internal Medicine. 15 July 1998; Volume 129: Issue 2: Pages 135-138

[107] Surks MI, Ocampo E. Subclinical thyroid disease. Am J Med. 1996; 100:217-23

[108] Staub JJ, Althaus BU, Engler H, Ryff AS, Trabucco P, Marquardt K, et al. Spectrum of subclinical and overt hypothyroidism: effect on thyrotropin, prolactin, and thyroid reserve, and metabolic impact on peripheral target tissues. Am J Med. 1992; 92:631-41.

[109] Yildirimkaya M, Ozata M, Yilmaz K, Kilinc C, Gundogan MA, Kutluay T. Lipoprotein(a) concentration in subclinical hypothyroidism before and after levo-thyroxine therapy. Endocr J. 1996; 43:731-6.

[110] Bunevicius R, Kazanavicius G, Zalinkevicius R, Prange AJ Jr. Effects of thyroxine as compared with thyroxine plus triiodothyronine in patients with hypothyroidism. N Engl J Med. 1999 Feb 11;340(6):469-70.

[111] Barbara Baker "No BMD Loss With Thyroid Replacement Tx". OB/GYN News. Sept 1, 2000. FindArticles.com. 09 Oct. 2006.

[112] Kuijpens JL, Nyklictek I, Louwman MW, Weetman TA, Pop VJ, Coebergh JW. Hypothyroidism might be related to breast cancer in post-menopausal women. Thyroid. 2005 Nov;15(11):1253-9.

[113] Garrison RL, Breeding PC. A metabolic basis for fibromyalgia and its related disorders: the possible role of resistance to thyroid hormone. Med Hypotheses. 2003 Aug;61(2):182-9.

[114] Beck-Peccoz P, Mannavola D, Persani L. Syndromes of thyroid hormone resistance. Ann Endocrinol (Paris). 2005 Jun;66(3):264-9.

[115] Tjorve E, Tjorve KM, Olsen JO, Senum R, Oftebro H. On commonness and rarity of thyroid hormone resistance: A discussion based on mechanisms of reduced sensitivity in peripheral tissues. Med Hypotheses. 2007 Mar 23.

[116] [no author listed] What is Subclinical Hypothyroidism? Medical Crossfire. December 2000; Vol 2, No 12.

[117] Feart C, Pallet V, Boucheron C, Higueret D, Alfos S, Letenneur L, Dartigues JF, Higueret P. Aging affects the retinoic acid and the triiodothyronine nuclear receptor mRNA expression in human peripheral blood mononuclear cells. Eur J Endocrinol. 2005 Mar;152(3):449-58.

[118] Takashi Akamizu, Leonard D. Kohn, Hitomi Hiratani, Misa Saijo, Kazuo Tahara and Kazuwa Nakao. Special Articles: Hashimoto's Thyroiditis with Heterogeneous Antithyrotropin Receptor Antibodies: Unique Epitopes May Contribute to the Regulation of Thyroid Function by the Antibodies1. The Journal of Clinical Endocrinology & Metabolism Vol. 85, No. 6 2116-2121. Copyright © 2000 by The Endocrine Society.

[119] Brucker-Davis F, Skarulis MC, Grace MB, Benichou J, Hauser P, Wiggs E, et al. Genetic and clinical features of 42 kindreds with resistance to thyroid hormone. The National Institutes of Health Prospective Study. Ann Intern Med. 1995; 123:572-83.

[120] Durrant-Peatfield B. Thyroid and adrenal dysfunction: the diagnosis and treatment of an endemic syndrome. Institute for Complementary Medicine, February 2006 Edition.

[121] Noth RH, Mazzaferri EL. Age and the endocrine system. Clin Geriatr Med. 1985 Feb;1(1):223-50.

[122] Knobel M, Medeiros-Neto G. An Outline of Inherited Disorders of the Thyroid Hormone Generating System. Thyroid 13(8):771-801, 2003. © 2003 Mary Ann Liebert, Inc.

[123] Burman, KD. Clinical Management of Hypothyroidism. [online] Available on Medscape® at /www.medscape.com/viewprogram/706. Accessed 2006 Sep 8.

[124] Burman, KD. Clinical Management of Hypothyroidism. [online] Available on Medscape at /www.medscape.com/viewprogram/706. Accessed 2006 Sep 8.

[125] Ghafoor F, Mansoor M, Malik T, Malik MS, Khan AU, Edwards R, Akhtar W. Role of thyroid peroxidase antibodies in the outcome of pregnancy. J Coll Physicians Surg Pak. 2006 Jul;16(7):468-71.

[126] Burman, KD. Clinical Management of Hypothyroidism: Thyroid Hormone Resistance. [online] Available on Medscape® at /www.medscape.com/viewprogram/706. Accessed 2006 Sep 9.

[127] Chatterjee VK. Resistance to thyroid hormone, and peroxisome-proliferator-activated receptor gamma resistance. Biochem Soc Trans. 2001; 29(Pt 2):227-31 (ISSN: 0300-5127).

[128] Rezvani I., DiGeorge AM, Dowshen SA, Bourdony CJ. Action of human growth hormone (hGH) on extrathyroidal conversion of thyroxine (T4) to triiodothyronine (T3) in children with hypopituitarism. Pediatric Research, Vol 15, 6-9, Copyright © 1981 by International Pediatric Research Foundation.

[129] De Groot, Leslie J. M.D., Georg Hennemann, M.D., Thyroid Manager, December 2002. http://www.thyroidmanager.org/Chapter6/Ch-6-3.htm.

[130] Fazio S, Palmieri EA, Lombardi G, Biondi B. Effects of thyroid hormone on the cardiovascular system. Recent Prog Horm Res. 2004;59:31-50.

[131] De Groot, Leslie J. M.D., Georg Hennemann, M.D., Thyroid Manager, December 2002. http://www.thyroidmanager.org/Chapter6/Ch-6-3.htm

[132] Bianchi G, Solaroli E, Zaccheroni V, Grossi G, Bargossi AM, Melchionda N, Marchesini G. Oxidative stress and anti-oxidant metabolites in patients with hyperthyroidism: effect of treatment. Horm Metab Res. 1999 Nov;31(11):620-4.

[133] Morkin E; Ladenson P; Goldman S; Adamson C. Thyroid hormone analogs for treatment of hypercholesterolemia and heart failure: past, present and future prospects. J Mol Cell Cardiol. 2004; 37(6):1137-46 (ISSN: 0022-2828).

[134] Morkin E; Ladenson P; Goldman S; Adamson C. Thyroid hormone analogs for treatment of hypercholesterolemia and heart failure: past, present and future prospects. J Mol Cell Cardiol. 2004; 37(6):1137-46 (ISSN: 0022-2828).

[135] Danzi S, Klein I. Thyroid hormone and the cardiovascular system. Minerva Endocrinol. 2004 Sep;29(3):139-50.

[136] Barbara Baker "No BMD Loss With Thyroid Replacement Tx". OB/GYN News. Sept 1, 2000. FindArticles.com. 09 Oct. 2006.

[137] Wartofsky L, Van Nostrand D, Burman KD. Overt and 'subclinical' hypothyroidism in women. Obstet Gynecol Surv. 2006 Aug;61(8):535-42.

[138] Miller KJ, Parsons TD, Whybrow PC, van Herle K, Rasgon N, van Herle A, Martinez D, Silverman DH, Bauer M. Memory improvement with treatment of hypothyroidism. Int J Neurosci. 2006 Aug;116(8):895-906.

[139] Friesema EC, Jansen J, Visser TJ. Thyroid hormone transporters. Biochem Soc Trans. 2005 Feb;33(Pt 1):228-32.

[140] Bianchi G, Solaroli E, Zaccheroni V, Grossi G, Bargossi AM, Melchionda N, Marchesini G. Oxidative stress and anti-oxidant metabolites in patients with hyperthyroidism: effect of treatment. Horm Metab Res. 1999 Nov;31(11):620-4.

[141] Freake HC; Govoni KE; Guda K; Huang C; Zinn SA. Actions and interactions of thyroid hormone and zinc status in growing rats. J Nutr. 2001; 131(4):1135-41 (ISSN: 0022-3166).

[142] Danzi S; Klein I. Thyroid hormone and the cardiovascular system. Minerva Endocrinol. 2004; 29(3):139-50 (ISSN: 0391-1977).

[143] Danzi S, Klein I. Thyroid hormone and the cardiovascular system. Minerva Endocrinol. 2004

Sep;29(3):139-50.

[144] Kovacs, P. Recurrent Pregnancy Loss. [online] Available at www.medscape.com/viewprogram/5293_pnt. Accessed 2006 Oct 13. Copyright © 2006 Medscape.

[145] Ables AZ, Baughman OL 3rd. Antidepressants: update on new agents and indications. Am Fam Physician. 2003 Feb 1;67(3):547-54.

[146] Bunevicius R, Kazanavicius G, Zalinkevicius R, Prange AJ Jr. Effects of thyroxine as compared with thyroxine plus triiodothyronine in patients with hypothyroidism. N Engl J Med. 1999 Feb 11;340(6):424-9.

[147] McGrath PJ, Quitkin FM, Klein DF. Bromocriptine treatment of relapses seen during selective serotonin re-uptake inhibitor treatment of depression [letter]. J Clin Psychopharmacol. 1995;15:289-291.

[148] Pallotti S, Gasbarrone A, Franzese IT. [Relationship between insulin secretion, and thyroid and ovary function in patients suffering from polycystic ovary][Article in Italian] Minerva Endocrinol. 2005 Sep;30(3):193-7.

[149] Gerwin RD. A review of myofascial pain and fibromyalgia--factors that promote their persistence. Acupunct Med. 2005 Sep;23(3):121-34.

[150] Smallridge RC. Disclosing subclinical thyroid disease. An approach to mild laboratory abnormalities and vague or absent symptoms. Postgrad Med. 2000 Jan;107(1):143-6, 149-52.

[151] Miller KJ, Parsons TD, Whybrow PC, van Herle K, Rasgon N, van Herle A, Martinez D, Silverman DH, Bauer M. Memory improvement with treatment of hypothyroidism. Int J Neurosci. 2006 Aug;116(8):895-906.

[152] Oerbeck B, Sundet K, Kase BF, Heyerdahl S. Congenital hypothyroidism: no adverse effects of high dose thyroxine treatment on adult memory, attention, and behaviour. Arch Dis Child. 2005 Feb;90(2):132-7.

[153] Garrison RL, Breeding PC. A metabolic basis for fibromyalgia and its related disorders: the possible role of resistance to thyroid hormone. Med Hypotheses. 2003 Aug;61(2):182-9.

[154] Rubin, AL. Subclinical Hypothyroidism. Medical Crossfire, Peer Exchange. December 2000. Available online at /www.medicalcrossfire.com.

[155] Bunevicius R, Jakubonien N, Jurkevicius R, Cernicat J, Lasas L, Prange AJ Jr. Thyroxine vs thyroxine plus triiodothyronine in treatment of hypothyroidism after thyroidectomy for Graves' disease. Endocrine. 2002 Jul;18(2):129-33.

[156] [no author listed] [online] Available at www.clinicaltrials.gov/ct/show/NCT00106119. Accessed 2006 Oct 13.

[157] Jaffiol C, Baldet L, Torresani J, Bismuth J, Papachristou C. A case of hypersensitivity to thyroid hormones with normally functioning thyroid gland and increased nuclear triiodothyronine receptors. J Endocrinol Invest. 1990 Nov;13(10):839-45. Jaffiol C, Baldet L, Torresani J, Bismuth J, Papachristou C. A case of hypersensitivity to thyroid hormones with normally functioning thyroid gland and increased nuclear triiodothyronine receptors. J Endocrinol Invest. 1990 Nov;13(10):839-45.

[158] Rubin, AL. Subclinical Hypothyroidism. Medical Crossfire, Peer Exchange. December 2000. Available online at /www.medicalcrossfire.com.

[159] Alevizaki M, Mantzou E, Cimponeriu AT, Alevizaki CC, Koutras DA. TSH may not be a good marker for adequate thyroid hormone replacement therapy. Wien Klin Wochenschr. 2005 Sep;117(18):636-40.

[160] Danzi S, Klein I. Potential uses of T3 in the treatment of human disease. Clin Cornerstone. 2005;7 Suppl 2:S9-15.

[161] Danzi S, Klein I. Potential uses of T3 in the treatment of human disease. Clin Cornerstone. 2005;7 Suppl 2:S9-15.

[162] Brucker-Davis F, Skarulis MC, Grace MB, Benichou J, Hauser P, Wiggs E, et al. Genetic and clinical features of 42 kindreds with resistance to thyroid hormone. The National Institutes of Health Prospective Study. Ann Intern Med. 1995; 123:572-83.

[163] Olivieri O, Girelli D, Stanzial AM, Rossi L, Bassi A, Corrocher R. Selenium, zinc, and thyroid hormones in healthy subjects: low T3/T4 ratio in the elderly is related to impaired selenium status. Biol Trace Elem Res. 1996 Jan;51(1):31-41.

[164] Santos GM, Pantoja CJ, Costa E Silva A, Rodrigues MC, Ribeiro RC, Simeoni LA, Lomri N, Neves FA. Thyroid hormone receptor binding to DNA and T3-dependent transcriptional activation are inhibited by uremic toxins.Nucl Recept. 2005 Apr 4;3(1):1.

[165] Oerbeck B, Sundet K, Kase BF, Heyerdahl S. Congenital hypothyroidism: no adverse effects of high dose thyroxine treatment on adult memory, attention, and behaviour. Arch Dis Child. 2005 Feb;90(2):132-

7.

[166] Bunevicius R, Jakubonien N, Jurkevicius R, Cernicat J, Lasas L, Prange AJ Jr. Thyroxine vs thyroxine plus triiodothyronine in treatment of hypothyroidism after thyroidectomy for Graves' disease. Endocrine. 2002 Jul;18(2):129-33.

[167] Bindi M, Pinelli M, Rosada J, Castiglioni M. [Atrial fibrillation and thyroid gland][Article in Italian] Recenti Prog Med. 2005 Nov;96(11):548-51.

[168] Trivieri MG, Oudit GY, Sah R, Kerfant BG, Sun H, Gramolini AO, Pan Y, Wickenden AD, Croteau W, Morreale de Escobar G, Pekhletski R, St Germain D, Maclennan DH, Backx PH. Cardiac-specific elevations in thyroid hormone enhance contractility and prevent pressure overload-induced cardiac dysfunction. Proc Natl Acad Sci U S A. 2006 Apr 11;103(15):6043-8.

[169] Olivieri O, Girelli D, Stanzial AM, Rossi L, Bassi A, Corrocher R. Selenium, zinc, and thyroid hormones in healthy subjects: low T3/T4 ratio in the elderly is related to impaired selenium status. Biol Trace Elem Res. 1996 Jan;51(1):31-41.

[170] Zimmermann MB, Bridson J, Bozo M, Grimci L, Selimaj V, Tanner MS. Severe iodine deficiency in southern Albania. Int J Vitam Nutr Res. 2003 Oct;73(5):347-50.

[171] Liberopoulos EN, Elisaf MS. Dyslipidemia in patients with thyroid disorders. Hormones (Athens). 2002 Oct-Dec;1(4):218-23.

[172] Vlase H, Lungu G, Vlase L. Cardiac disturbances in thyrotoxicosis: diagnosis, incidence, clinical features and management. Endocrinologie. 1991;29(3-4):155-60.

[173] Kalmijn S, Mehta KM, Pols HA, Hofman A, Drexhage HA, Breteler MM 2000 Subclinical hyperthyroidism and the risk of dementia: The Rotterdam Study. Clin Endocrinol (Oxf) 53:733–737.

[174] Wald DA, Silver A. Cardiovascular manifestations of thyroid storm: a case report. J Emerg Med. 2003 Jul;25(1):23-8.

[175] Hulley S, Grady D, Bush T, et al. Randomized trial of estrogen plus progestin for secondary prevention of coronary heart disease in postmenopausal women: Heart and Estrogen/progestin Replacement Study (HERS) Research Group. JAMA 1998;280:605-613.

[176] [no author listed] Findings from the WHI Postmenopausal Hormone Therapy Trials. Available online at www.nhlbi.nih.gov/whi/. Accessed 2006 Sep 10.

[177] Rossi R; Bursi F; Veronesi B; Cagnacci A; Modena MG. Effects of progestins on estrogen-induced increase in C-reactive protein in postmenopausal women. Maturitas. 2004; 49(4):315-20 (ISSN: 0378-5122).

[178] Campagnoli C, Ambroggio S, Biglia N, Sismondi P. Conjugated estrogens and breast cancer risk. Gynecol Endocrinol. 1999 Dec;13 Suppl 6:13-9.

[179] Albertazzi P, et al. Dietary Soy Supplementation and Phytoestrogen Levels. Obstet Gynecol. 94 (2): 229. Copyright © 1999 by The American College of Obstetricians and Gynecologists. Published by Elsevier Science Inc.

[180] Hargrove JT, Maxson WS, Wentz AC, Burnett LS. Menopausal hormone replacement therapy with continuous daily oral micronized estradiol and progesterone. Obstet Gynecol. 1989 Apr;73(4):606-12.

[181] Hargrove, JT; Osteen, KC. An Alternative Method of Hormone Replacement Therapy Using the Natural Sex Steroids. Infertility and Reproductive Medicine Clinics of North America. Volume 6, Number 4, October 1995.

[182] Hargrove, JT; Osteen, KC. An Alternative Method of Hormone Replacement Therapy Using the Natural Sex Steroids. Infertility and Reproductive Medicine Clinics of North America. Volume 6, Number 4, October 1995.

[183] Shimizu Y. [Article in Japanese] [Estrogen: estrone (E1), estradiol (E2), estriol (E3) and estetrol (E4)] Nippon Rinsho. 2005 Aug;63 Suppl 8:425-38.

[184] Hunt CM, Westerkam WR, Stave GM. Effect of age and gender on the activity of human hepatic CYP3A. Biochem Pharmacol 1992;44:275-83.

[185] Robb-Nicholson C. By the way, doctor. In the lead article about HRT use in your April issue, you didn't mention Estrace. I've taken it for several years, without any problems. But am I getting the same benefits as I would with Premarin, and are the risks similar? Harv Womens Health Watch. 2000; 8(2):8 (ISSN: 1070-910X).

[186] Apgar, B. Gallbladder Disease in Women Receiving ERT - estrogen replacement therapy - Brief Article. American Family Physician. Nov 1, 2000.

[187] Psaty, BM et al. Hormone Replacement Therapy, Prothrombotic Mutations, and the Risk of Incident

Nonfatal Myocardial Infarction in Postmenopausal Women. JAMA. 2001;285:906-913.

[188] Psaty, BM et al. Hormone Replacement Therapy, Prothrombotic Mutations, and the Risk of Incident Nonfatal Myocardial Infarction in Postmenopausal Women. JAMA. 2001;285:906-913.

[189] Baker VL. Alternatives to Oral Estrogen Therapy. Obstetrics and Gynecology Clinics of North America, Vol. 21, No. 2, June 1994, pp. 271-97.

[190] Scarabin PY, et al. Differential association of oral and transdermal oestrogen-replacement therapy with venous thrombonembolism risk. The Lancet 2003; 362:428-432.

[191] Baker VL. Alternatives to Oral Estrogen Therapy. Obstetrics and Gynecology Clinics of North America, Vol. 21, No. 2, June 1994, pp. 271-97

[192] Psaty, BM et al. Hormone Replacement Therapy, Prothrombotic Mutations, and the Risk of Incident Nonfatal Myocardial Infarction in Postmenopausal Women. JAMA. 2001;285:906-913.

[193] Cobin, Rh. HRT and Cardiocascular Protection (January 2001 -- Live Event). Medical Crossfire, June 2001; Vol. 3 [6]: 139-40.

[194] Worcester S. Young, Healthy HRT Users at Low Risk for CV Event: WHI results may not apply to healthy women treating menopausal symptoms. Family Practice News, Volume 33, Issue 11, Pages 1-2 (June 2003).

[195] Dubey RK, Imthurn B, Barton M, Jackson EK. Vascular consequences of menopause and hormone therapy: importance of timing of treatment and type of estrogen. Cardiovasc Res. 2005 May 1;66(2):295-306.

[196] Hargrove JT, Eisenberg E. Menopause. Medical clinics of North America, 194 Nov; 79 (6); 1337-55.

[197] de Lignieres B, Vincens M. Differential effects of exogenous oestradiol and progesterone on mood in post-menopausal women: individual dose/effect relationship. Maturitas. 1982 Apr;4(1):67-72.

[198] Hargrove, JT; Osteen, KC. An Alternative Method of Hormone Replacement Therpay Using the Natural Sex Steroids. Infertility and Reproductive Medicine Clinics of North America. Volume 6, Number 4, October 1995.

[199] Furman RH. 1968. Are gonadal hormones (estrogens and androgens) of significance in the development of ischemic heart disease. Ann NY Sci 149:822–833.

[200] Thacker, HL. Update on Hormone Replacement: Sorting Out the Options for Preventing Coronary Artery Disease and Osteoporosis. Medscape General Medicine 1(1), 1999. © 1999 Medscape. Available online at www.medscape.com/viewarticle/408802.

[201] Thacker, HL. Update on Hormone Replacement: Sorting Out the Options for Preventing Coronary Artery Disease and Osteoporosis. Medscape General Medicine 1(1), 1999. © 1999 Medscape. Available online at www.medscape.com/viewarticle/408802.

[202] Thacker, HL. Update on Hormone Replacement: Sorting Out the Options for Preventing Coronary Artery Disease and Osteoporosis. Medscape General Medicine 1(1), 1999. © 1999 Medscape. Available online at www.medscape.com/viewarticle/408802.

[203] Thacker, HL. Update on Hormone Replacement: Sorting Out the Options for Preventing Coronary Artery Disease and Osteoporosis. Medscape General Medicine 1(1), 1999. © 1999 Medscape. Available online at www.medscape.com/viewarticle/408802.

[204] Hall G, Phillips TJ. J Am Acad Dermatol. 2005 Oct;53(4):555-68; quiz 569-72. Estrogen and skin: the effects of estrogen, menopause, and hormone replacement therapy on the skin.

[205] Hall G, Phillips TJ. J Am Acad Dermatol. 2005 Oct;53(4):555-68; quiz 569-72. Estrogen and skin: the effects of estrogen, menopause, and hormone replacement therapy on the skin.

[206] Shepherd, JE. Effects of Estrogen on Cognition, Mood, and Degenerative Brain Diseases. J Am Pharm Assoc 41(2):221-228, 2001. © 2001 American Pharmaceutical Association.

[207] Shepherd, JE. Effects of Estrogen on Cognition, Mood, and Degenerative Brain Diseases. J Am Pharm Assoc 41(2):221-228, 2001. © 2001 American Pharmaceutical Association.

[208] Shepherd, JE. Effects of Estrogen on Cognition, Mood, and Degenerative Brain Diseases. J Am Pharm Assoc 41(2):221-228, 2001. © 2001 American Pharmaceutical Association.

[209] Doren M. Hormonal replacement regimens and bleeding. Maturitas. 2000 Jan;34 Suppl 1:S17-23.

[210] Grady D, Rubin SM, Pettiti DB, et al: Hormone replacement therapy to prevent disease and prolong life in postmenopausal women. Ann Intern Med 117:1016-1017, 1992.

[211] Thacker, HL. Update on Hormone Replacement: Sorting Out the Options for Preventing Coronary Artery Disease and Osteoporosis. Medscape General Medicine 1(1), 1999. © 1999 Medscape. Available online at www.medscape.com/viewarticle/408802.

[212] Taguchi A, Sanada M, Suei Y, Ohtsuka M, Nakamoto T, Lee K, Tsuda M, Ohama K, Tanimoto K, Bollen AM. Effect of estrogen use on tooth retention, oral bone height, and oral bone porosity in Japanese postmenopausal women. Menopause. 2004 Sep-Oct;11(5):556-62.

[213] McKuen BS, Alves BS. Estrogen action in the central nervous system. *Endocrin Rev*.1999;20:279-307.

[214] Haan MN, Klein R, Klein BE, Deng Y, Blythe LK, Seddon JM, Musch DC, Kuller LH, Hyman LG, Wallace RB. Hormone therapy and age-related macular degeneration: the Women's Health Initiative Sight Exam Study. Arch Ophthalmol. 2006 Jul;124(7):988-92.

[215] Klein BEK, Klein R, Ritter LL. Is there evidence of an estrogen effect on age-related lens opacities? Arch Ophthalmol. 1994;112:85-91.

[216] Shepherd, JE. Effects of Estrogen on Cognition, Mood, and Degenerative Brain Diseases. J Am Pharm Assoc 41(2):221-228, 2001. © 2001 American Pharmaceutical Association.

[217] Doren M. Hormonal replacement regimens and bleeding. Maturitas. 2000 Jan;34 Suppl 1:S17-23.

[218] Punnonen R, Vilska S, Rauramo L. Skinfold thickness and long-term post-menopausal hormone therapy. Maturitas. 1984 Apr;5(4):259-62.

[219] Stampfer MJ, Colditz GA. Estrogen replacement and coronary heart disease: a quantitative assessment of the epidemiologic evidence. Prev Med. 1991;20:47-63.

[220] Stampfer MJ, Colditz GA, Willett WC, Manson JE, Rosner B, Speizer FE, Hennekens CH. Postmenopausal estrogen therapy and cardiovascular disease. Ten-year follow-up from the nurses' health study. N Engl J Med. 1991 Sep 12;325(11):756-62.

[221] [no author listed] NHBLI NIH NEWS. WHI Study Finds No Heart Disease Benefit, Increased Stroke Risk With Estrogen Alone. Tuesday, April 13, 2004, 4:00 p.m. ET. [online] Available at www.nhlbi.nih.gov/whi. Accessed 2006 Oct 7.

[222] Chen H ; Chen Y ; Tian W ; Lei S ; Peng R. [Effects of estradiol and isoflavoid on the expression of adhesion molecules on neutrophils] Hua Xi Yi Ke Da Xue Xue Bao. 2001; 32(1):27-31 (ISSN: 0257-7712).

[223] Wise PM; Dubal DB; Wilson ME; Rau SW; Böttner M. Minireview: neuroprotective effects of estrogen-new insights into mechanisms of action. Endocrinology. 2001; 142(3):969-73 (ISSN: 0013-7227).

[224] Shoupe D. Hormone replacement therapy: reassessing the risks and benefits. Hosp Pract (Minneap). 1999 Aug 15;34(8):97-103, 107-8, 113-4.

[225] Shoupe D. Hormone replacement therapy: reassessing the risks and benefits. Hosp Pract (Minneap). 1999 Aug 15;34(8):97-103, 107-8, 113-4.

[226] Shoupe D. Hormone replacement therapy: reassessing the risks and benefits. Hosp Pract (Minneap). 1999 Aug 15;34(8):97-103, 107-8, 113-4.

[227] Meisler, JG. Toward Optimal Health: The Experts Provide a Current Perspective on Perimenopause. J Womens Health 12(7):609-615, 2003. © 2003 Mary Ann Liebert, Inc.

[228] Dupont WD, Page DL: Menopausal, estrogen replacement therapy, and breast cancer. Arch Intern Med 151:67-72, 1991.

[229] Effects of hormone replacement therapy on endometrial histology in postmenopausal women. The Postmenopausal Estrogen/Progestin Interventions (PEPI) Trial. The Writing Group for the PEPI Trial. JAMA. 1996;275:370-375.

[230] [no author listed] Findings from the WHI Postmenopausal Hormone Therapy Trials. Available online at www.nhlbi.nih.gov/whi/. Accessed 2006 Sep 10.

[231] Meisler, JG. Toward Optimal Health: The Experts Provide a Current Perspective on Perimenopause. J Womens Health 12(7):609-615, 2003. © 2003 Mary Ann Liebert, Inc.

[232] Prior JC, Vigna Y, Sciarretta D, et al. Conditioning exercise decreases premenstrual symptoms: a prospective, controlled 6-month trial. *Fertil Steril*. 1987;47:402-8.

[233] Wolanske, KA; Gordon, RL. Uterine Artery Embolization: Where Does it Stand in the Management of Uterine Leiomyomas? Part 2. Appl Radiol 33(10):18-25, 2004. © 2004 Anderson Publishing, Ltd.

[234] Fettes I. Migraine in the menopause. Neurology. 1999;53 (suppl 1):S29-S33.

[235] Walsh BW, Kuller LH, Wild RA, et al. Effects of raloxifene on serum lipids and coagulation factors in healthy postmenopausal women. JAMA. 1998;2790:1445-1451.

[236] Hulley S, Grady D, Bush T, et al. Randomized trial of estrogen plus progestin for secondary prevention of coronary heart disease in postmenopausal women: Heart and Estrogen/progestin Replacement Study (HERS) Research Group. JAMA 1998;280:605-613.

[237] Birkenfeld L, Yemini M, Kase NG, et al. Menopause-related oral alveolar bone resorption: a review of relatively unexplored consequences of estrogen deficiency. Menopause. 1999;6:129-133.

[238] Freeman EW, et al. Associations of hormones and menopausal status with depressed mood in women with no history of depression. Arch Gen Psychiatry April 2006;63:375-82.

[239] Campagnoli C; Colombo P; De Aloysio D; Gambacciani M; Grazioli I; Nappi C; Serra GB; Genazzani AR. Positive effects on cardiovascular and breast metabolic markers of oral estradiol and dydrogesterone in comparison with transdermal estradiol and norethisterone acetate. Maturitas. 2002; 41(4):299-311 (ISSN: 0378-5122).

[240] Bastian LA, Smith CM, Nanda K. Is this woman perimenopausal? JAMA. 2003 Feb 19;289(7):895-902.

[241] Dalal, S; Zhukovsky, DS. Pathoilable online at physiology and Management of Hot Flashes. www.SupportiveOncology.net; VOLUME 4, NUMBER 7; JULY/AUGUST 2006. Available online at www.SupportiveOncology.net.

[242] Freedman RR, Norton D, Woodward S, et al. Core body temperature and circadian rhythm of hot flashes in menopausal women. J Clin Endocrinol Metab 1995;80:2354-2358.

[243] Cho JJ, Cadet P, Salamon E, Mantione K, Stefano GB. The nongenomic protective effects of estrogen on the male cardiovascular system: clinical and therapeutic implications in aging men. Med Sci Monit. 2003 Mar;9(3):RA63-8.

[244] Bracco GL, Carli P, Sonni L, Maestrini G, De Marco A, Taddei GL, Cattaneo A. Clinical and histologic effects of topical treatments of vulval lichen sclerosus. A critical evaluation. J Reprod Med. 1993 Jan;38(1):37-40.

[245] Leiblum S, Bachmann GA, Kemmann E, Colburn D, Swartzman L. Vaginal atrophy and the postmenopausal woman: the importance of sexual activity and hormones. JAMA 1983;249:2195-8.

[246] Kightlinger, RS. Menopause Matters. Vaginal Atrophy: Clinical Evaluation and Management. Available online at http://www.femalepatient.com/html/arc/sig/meno/articles/030_04_065.asp. Accessed March 19, 2007.

[247] Cobin, Rh. HRT and Cardiocascular Protection (January 2001 -- Live Event). Medical Crossfire, June 2001; Vol. 3 [6]: 139-40.

[248] Psaty, BM et al. Hormone Replacement Therapy, Prothrombotic Mutations, and the Risk of Incident Nonfatal Myocardial Infarction in Postmenopausal Women. JAMA. 2001;285:906-913.

[249] Iqbal, MM. Osteoporosis: Epidemiology, Diagnosis, and Treatment. South Med J 93(1):2-18, 2000. © 2000 Southern Medical Association.

[250] Wachter, K. Treat the Very Elderly for Low Bone Density: Bone loss accelerates as patients age, yet 'we aren't doing a very good job' of treating the very elderly. Family Practice News, Volume 35, Issue 9, Page 67 (01 May 2005).

[251] Siris ES, Miller PD, Barrett-Connor E, Faulkner KG, Wehren LE, Abbott TA, Berger ML, Santora AC, Sherwood LM. Identification and fracture outcomes of undiagnosed low bone mineral density in postmenopausal women: results from the National Osteoporosis Risk Assessment. JAMA. 2001 Dec 12;286(22):2815-22.

[252] Davidson, MR. Pharmacotherapeutics for Osteoporosis Prevention and Treatment. J Midwifery Womens Health 48(1):39-54, 2003. © 2003 Elsevier Science, Inc.

[253] Villareal DT, Binder EF, Williams DB, Schechtman KB, Yarasheski KE, Kohrt WM. Bone mineral density response to estrogen replacement in frail elderly women: a randomized controlled trial. JAMA. 2001 Aug 15;286(7):815-20.

[254] Sipila S, Heikkinen E, Cheng S, Suominen H, Saari P, Kovanen V, Alen M, Rantanen T. Endogenous hormones, muscle strength, and risk of fall-related fractures in older women. J Gerontol A Biol Sci Med Sci. 2006 Jan;61(1):92-6.

[255] Lanham-New SA. Nutritional Influences on Bone Health: An Update on Current Research and Clinical Implications . [online] Available at www.medscape.com/viewprogram/5034_pnt.

[256] Adams J; Pepping J. Vitamin K in the Treatment and Prevention of Osteoporosis and Arterial Calcification. Am J Health-Syst Pharm. 2005;62(15):1574-1581. ©2005 American Society of Health-System Pharmacists.

[257] Adams J; Pepping J. Vitamin K in the Treatment and Prevention of Osteoporosis and Arterial Calcification. Am J Health-Syst Pharm. 2005;62(15):1574-1581. ©2005 American Society of Health-System Pharmacists.

[258] Cranney A, Wells G, et al; Osteoporosis Methodology Group and The Osteoporosis Research Advisory Group. Meta-analyses of therapies for postmenopausal osteoporosis. II. Meta-analysis of alendronate for the treatment of postmenopausal women. Endocr Rev. 2002 Aug;23(4):508-16.

[259] Davidson, MR. Pharmacotherapeutics for Osteoporosis Prevention and Treatment. J Midwifery Womens Health 48(1):39-54, 2003. © 2003 Elsevier Science, Inc.

[260] Quandt SA, Thompson DE, Schneider DL, Nevitt MC, Black DM. Effect of alendronate on vertebral fracture risk in women with bone mineral density T scores of -1.6 to -2.5 at the femoral neck: the Fracture Intervention Trial. Mayo Clin Proc March 2005;80:343-9.

[261] Schousboe JT, et al. Cost-effectiveness of alendronate therapy for osteopenic postmenopausal women. Ann Intern Med May 3, 2005;142:734-41.

[262] Ference, J.D.; Wilson, S.A. STEPS: Ibandronate (Boniva) for Treatment and Prevention of Osteoporosis in Postmenopausal Women. American Family Physician; January 15, 2006 (table of contents)
Vol. 73 No. 2:305-306.

[263] Ference, J.D.; Wilson, S.A. STEPS: Ibandronate (Boniva) for Treatment and Prevention of Osteoporosis in Postmenopausal Women. American Family Physician; January 15, 2006 (table of contents)
Vol. 73 No. 2:305-306.

[264] Bischoff-Ferrari HA, Willett WC, Wong JB, Giovannucci E, Dietrich T, Dawson-Hughes B. Fracture prevention with vitamin D supplementation: a meta-analysis of randomized controlled trials. JAMA 2005;293; 2257-64.

[265] Boonen S, Lips P, Bouillon R, Bischoff-Ferrari HA, Vanderschueren D, Haentjens P. Need for additional calcium to reduce the risk of hip fracture with vitamin D supplementation: evidence from a comparative meta-analysis of randomized controlled trials. J Clin Endocrinol Metab. 2007 Jan 30.

[266] Quandt SA; Thompson DE; Schneider DL; Nevitt MC; Black DM. Effect of alendronate on vertebral fracture risk in women with bone mineral density T scores of-1.6 to -2.5 at the femoral neck: the Fracture Intervention Trial. Mayo Clin Proc. 2005; 80(3):343-9 (ISSN: 0025-6196).

[267] Ishida Y, Kawai S. Comparative efficacy of hormone replacement therapy, etidronate, calcitonin, alfacalcidol, and vitamin K in postmenopausal women with osteoporosis: The Yamaguchi Osteoporosis Prevention Study. Am J Med. 2004 Oct 15;117(8):549-55.

[268] Sipila S, Heikkinen E, Cheng S, Suominen H, Saari P, Kovanen V, Alen M, Rantanen T. Endogenous hormones, muscle strength, and risk of fall-related fractures in older women. J Gerontol A Biol Sci Med Sci. 2006 Jan;61(1):92-6.

[269] Lanham-New SA. Nutritional Influences on Bone Health: An Update on Current Research and Clinical Implications . [online] Available at www.medscape.com/viewprogram/5034_pnt.

[270] Adams J; Pepping J. Vitamin K in the Treatment and Prevention of Osteoporosis and Arterial Calcification. Am J Health-Syst Pharm. 2005;62(15):1574-1581. ©2005 American Society of Health-System Pharmacists.

[271] Ross EA, Szabo NJ, Tebbett IR. Lead content of calcium supplements. JAMA. 2000 Sep 20;284(11):1425-9.

[272] Shah SV; Alam MG. Role of iron in atherosclerosis. Am J Kidney Dis. 2003; 41(3 Suppl 1):S80-3 (ISSN: 1523-6838).

[273] Valko M, Morris H, Cronin MT. Metals, toxicity and oxidative stress. Curr Med Chem. 2005;12(10):1161-208.

[274] New SA. Acid-base homeostasis in the skeleton: Is there a fruit and vegetable link to bone health? In: New SA, Bonjour JP, eds. Nutritional Aspects of Bone Health. Cambridge, UK: Royal Society of Chemistry; 2003: 291-311.

[275] Van Meurs JBJ, Dhonukshe-Rutten RAM, Pluijm SMF, et al. Homocysteine levels and the risk of osteoporotic fracture. N Engl J Med. 2004;350:2033-2041

[276] Hargrove, JT; Osteen, KC. An Alternative Method of Hormone Replacement Therpay Using the Natural Sex Steroids. Infertility and Reproductive Medicine Clinics of North America. Volume 6, Number 4, October 1995.

[277] [No authors listed] Medroxyprogesterone acetate. IARC Monogr Eval Carcinog Risk Chem Hum. 1979 Dec;21:417-29.

[278] Klaiber EL; Vogel W; Rako S. A critique of the Women's Health Initiative hormone therapy study. Fertil Steril. 2005; 84(6):1589-601 (ISSN: 1556-5653).

[279] Thomas T, Rhodin J, Clark L, Garces A. Progestins initiate adverse events of menopausal estrogen therapy. Climacteric. 2003 Dec;6(4):293-301.

[280] Campagnoli C, Clavel-Chapelon F, Kaaks R, Peris C, Berrino F. Progestins and progesterone in hormone replacement therapy and the risk of breast cancer. J Steroid Biochem Mol Biol. 2005 Jul;96(2):95-

108.

[281] Cushman M, Legault C, Barrett-Connor E, et al. Effect of postmenopausal hormones on inflammation-sensitive proteins: the Postmenopausal Estrogen/Progestin Interventions (PEPI) Study. Circulation. 1999;100:717-722.

[282] Clark MK, Sowers M, Levy B, Nichols S. Bone mineral density loss and recovery during 48 months in first-time users of depot medroxyprogesterone acetate. Fertil Steril. 2006 Nov;86(5):1466-74.

[283] Archer B, Irwin D, Jensen K, Johnson ME, Rorie J. Depot medroxyprogesterone. Management of side-effects commonly associated with its contraceptive use. J Nurse Midwifery. 1997 Mar-Apr;42(2):104-11.

[284] Klaiber EL; Vogel W; Rako S. A critique of the Women's Health Initiative hormone therapy study. Fertil Steril. 2005; 84(6):1589-601 (ISSN: 1556-5653).

[285] Simon JA. Micronized progesterone: vaginal and oral uses. Clin Obstet Gynecol 1995;38:902-14.

[286] Online at www.nlm.nih.gov/medlineplus/ency/article/003714.htm. Accessed 2006 Oct 12.

[287] Campagnoli C, Clavel-Chapelon F, Kaaks R, Peris C, Berrino F. Progestins and progesterone in hormone replacement therapy and the risk of breast cancer. J Steroid Biochem Mol Biol. 2005 Jul;96(2):95-108.

[288] Attia MA, Zayed I. Thirteen-weeks subcutaneous treatment with high dose of natural sex hormones in rats with special reference to their effect on the pituitary-gonadal axis. II. Progesterone. Dtsch Tierarztl Wochenschr. 1989 Oct;96(9):445-9.

[289] Effects of estrogen or estrogen/progestin regimens on heart disease risk factors in postmenopausal women. Writing Group for the PEPI Trial. JAMA. 1995;273:1389-96.

[290] Hargrove JT, Maxson WS, Wentz AC, Burnett LS. Menopausal hormone replacement therapy with continuous daily oral micronized estradiol and progesterone. Obstet Gynecol. 1989 Apr;73(4):606-12.

[291] Sitruk-Ware R, Bricaire C, DeLignieres B, et al. Oral Micronized progesterone. Bioavailability pharmacokinetics, pharmacological and therapeutic implications—A Review, Contraception. 1987; 36:373-402.

[292] WEN-SEN LEE, CHAO-WEI LIU, SHU-HUI JUAN, YU-CHIH LIANG, PEI-YIN HO, AND YI-HSUAN LEE. Molecular Mechanism of Progesterone-Induced
Antiproliferation in Rat Aortic Smooth Muscle Cells. Endocrinology 144(7):2785–2790. Copyright © 2003 by The Endocrine Society doi: 10.1210/en.2003-0045.

[293] McCrohon JA; Nakhla S; Jessup W; Stanley KK; Celermajer DS. Estrogen and progesterone reduce lipid accumulation in human monocyte-derived macrophages: a sex-specific effect. Circulation. 1999; 100(23):2319-25 (ISSN: 0009-7322).

[294] Campagnoli C, Clavel-Chapelon F, aaks R, Peris C, Berrino F. Progestins and progesterone in hormone replacement therapy and the risk of breast cancer. J Steroid Biochem Mol Biol. 2005 Jul;96(2):95-108.

[295] Lydeking-Olsen E, Beck-Jensen JE, Setchell KD, Holm-Jensen T.
Soymilk or progesterone for prevention of bone loss--a 2 year randomized, placebo-controlled trial. Eur J Nutr. 2004 Aug;43(4):246-57.

[296] Randall TC, Kurman RJ. Progestin treatment of atypical hyperplasia and well-differentiated carcinoma of the endometrium in women under age 40. Obstet Gynecol 1997;90:434-40.

[297] Fraser IS. Regulating menstrual bleeding. A prime function of progesterone. J Reprod Med 1999;44(2 suppl):158-64.

[298] Arafat ES, Hargrove JT, Maxson WS, Desiderio DM, Wentz AC, Andersen RN. Sedative and hypnotic effects of oral administration of micronized progesterone may be mediated through its metabolites. Am J Obstet Gynecol. 1988 Nov;159(5):1203-9.

[299] Vanselow W, Dennerstein L, Greenwood KM, de Lignieres B. Effect of progesterone and its 5 alpha and 5 beta metabolites on symptoms of premenstrual syndrome according to route of administration. J Psychosom Obstet Gynaecol. 1996 Mar;17(1):29-38.

[300] Maxson WS. The use of progesterone in the treatment of PMS. Clin Obstet Gynecol. 1987:30:465-477

[301] Ahlgrimm, M. (May 2003). Managing pms and perimenopause symptoms The role of compounded medications, Advance for Nurse Practitioners, (11)5, p. 53.

[302] APGAR, B.S., GREENBERG, G. Practical Therapeutics Using Progestins in Clinical Practice. AFP - October 15, 2000.

[303] Fitzpatrick, LA; Pace, C; Wiita, B. Comparison of Regimens Containing Oral Micronized Progesterone or Medroxyprogesterone Acetate on Quality of Life in Postmenopausal Women: A Cross-Sectional Survey. Journal of Women's Health & Gender-Based Medicine. May 2000, Vol. 9, No. 4 :381 -387.

304 Davis SR, Guay AT, Shifren JL, Mazer NA. Endocrine aspects of female sexual dysfunction. J Sex Med. 2004 Jul;1(1):82-6.

305 Hargrove JT, Maxson WS, Wentz AC, Burnett LS. Menopausal hormone replacement therapy with continuous daily oral micronized estradiol and progesterone. Obstet Gynecol. 1989:73: 606-612.

306 Zumpe D, Clancy AN, Michael RP. Progesterone decreases mating and estradiol uptake in preoptic areas of male monkeys. Physiol Behav. 2001 Nov-Dec;74(4-5):603-12.

307 O'Leary P, Feddema P, Chan K, Taranto M, Smith M, Evans S. Salivary, but not serum or urinary levels of progesterone are elevated after topical application of progesterone cream to pre-and postmenopausal women. Clin Endocrinol (Oxf). 2000 Nov;53(5):615-20.

308 Berek JS, Hacker NF, eds. Practical gynecologic oncology. 2d ed. Baltimore: Williams & Wilkins, 1994:285-326, with information from Karlsson B, Granberg S, Wikland M, Ylostalto P, Torvid K, Marsal K, et al. Transvaginal ultrasonography of the endometrium in women with postmenopausal bleeding: a Nordic multicenter study. Am J Obstet Gynecol 1995;172:1488-94.

309 Chudnoff, SG. Ask the Experts about Gynecology and Reproductive Endocrinology. From Medscape Ob/Gyn & Women's Health. Endometrial Hyperplasia. [online] Available at www.medscape.com/viewarticle/507187. Accessed 2006 Oct 12.

310 Berek JS, Hacker NF, eds. Practical gynecologic oncology. 2d ed. Baltimore: Williams & Wilkins, 1994:285-326, with information from Karlsson B, Granberg S, Wikland M, Ylostalto P, Torvid K, Marsal K, et al. Transvaginal ultrasonography of the endometrium in women with postmenopausal bleeding: a Nordic multicenter study. Am J Obstet Gynecol 1995;172:1488-94.

311 Goldstein SR, Zeltser I, Horan CK, Snyder JR, Schwartz LB. Ultrasonography-based triage for perimenopausal patients with abnormal uterine bleeding. Am J Obstet Gynecol 1997; 177: 102-8.

312 Wachter, K. UAE Shows Some Advantage Over Myomectomy. Family Practie News, Volume 35, Issue 5, Page 59 (01 March 2005).

313 Walker WJ, McDowell SJ. Pregnancy After Uterine Artery Embolization for Leiomyomata: a Series of 56 Completed Pregnancies. Am J Obstet Gynecol. 2006;195:1266-1271.

314 [no authors listed] U.S. Preventive Services Task Force. Screening for Cervical Cancer. Release Date: January 2003. Available online at www.ahrq.gov/clinic/uspstf/uspscerv.htm. Accessed 2006 Oct 12.

315 [no authors listed] U.S. Preventive Services Task Force. Screening for Breast Cancer. Release Date: February 2002. Available online at www.ahrq.gov/clinic/uspstf/uspsbrca.htm. Accessed 2006 Oct 12.

316 Wren BG, Day RO, McLachlan AJ, Williams KM. Pharmacokinetics of estradiol, progesterone, testosterone and dehydroepiandrosterone after transbuccal administration to postmenopausal women. Climacteric. 2003 Jun;6(2):104-11.

317 Warren MP, Shantha S. Uses of progesterone in clinical practice. Int J Fertil Womens Med. 1999 Mar-Apr;44(2):96-103.

318 Bitran, D.; Shiekh, M.; McLeod, M. Anxiolytic Effect of Progesterone is Mediated by the Neurosteroid Allopregnanolone at Brain GABAA Receptors. Journal of Neuroendocrinology, Volume 7 Page 171 - March 1995 doi:10.1111/j.1365-2826.1995.tb00744.x, Volume 7, Issue 3.

319 Simon JA. Micronized progesterone: vaginal and oral uses. Clin Obstet Gynecol 1995;38:902-14.

320 Zitzmann M; Erren M; Kamischke A; Simoni M; Nieschlag E. Endogenous progesterone and the exogenous progestin norethisterone enanthate are associated with a proinflammatory profile in healthy men. J Clin Endocrinol Metab. 2005; 90(12):6603-8 (ISSN: 0021-972X).

321 Hargrove, J, Osteen, K. An alternative method of hormone replacement therapy using the natural sex steroids. *Infertility and Reproductive Medicine Clinics of North America* 1995;4:653-74.

322 Hargrove JT, Maxson WS, Wentz AC, Burnett LS. Menopausal hormone replacement therapy with continuous daily oral micronized estradiol and progesterone. Obstet Gynecol. 1989 Apr;73(4):606-12.

323 Hargrove JT, Maxson WS, Wentz AC, Burnett LS. Menopausal hormone replacement therapy with continuous daily oral micronized estradiol and progesterone. Obstet Gynecol. 1989 Apr;73(4):606-12.

324 Rubin, R. Out of the hot flash and into the fire. USA TODAY. [online] Available at www.usatoday.com/news/health/2005-03-29-menopause_x.htm.

325 Chudnoff, SG. Ask the Experts about Gynecology and Reproductive Endocrinology. From Medscape Ob/Gyn & Women's Health. Endometrial Hyperplasia. [online] Available at www.medscape.com/viewarticle/507187. Accessed 2006 Oct 12.

326 Ng AB, Reagan JW, Hawliczek S, Wentz BW. Significance of endometrial cells in the detection of endometrial carcinoma and its precursors. Acta Cytol 1974;18:356-61.

[327] O'Leary P, Feddema P, Chan K, Taranto M, Smith M, Evans S. Salivary, but not serum or urinary levels of progesterone are elevated after topical application of progesterone cream to pre-and postmenopausal women. Clin Endocrinol (Oxf). 2000 Nov;53(5):615-20.

[328] Savine R, Sonksen P. Growth hormone - hormone replacement for the somatopause? Horm Res. 2000;53 Suppl 3:37-41.

[329] Melton LJ 3rd, Khosla S, Riggs BL. Epidemiology of sarcopenia. Mayo Clin Proc. 2000 Jan;75 Suppl:S10-2; discussion S12-3.

[330] Colao, A; di Somma, C; et al. Improved Cardiovascular Risk Factors and Cardiac Performance after 12 Months of Growth Hormone (GH) Replacement in Young Adult Patients with GH Deficiency. The Journal of Clinical Endocrinology & Metabolism Vol. 86, No. 5 1874-1881. Copyright © 2001 by The Endocrine Society.

[331] Volterrani M, Desenzani P, Lorusso R, d'Aloia A, Manelli F, Giustina A. Haemodynamic effects of intravenous growth hormone in congestive heart failure. Lancet 1997;349:1067-8.

[332] Colao, A; di Somma, C; et al. Improved Cardiovascular Risk Factors and Cardiac Performance after 12 Months of Growth Hormone (GH) Replacement in Young Adult Patients with GH Deficiency. The Journal of Clinical Endocrinology & Metabolism Vol. 86, No. 5 1874-1881. Copyright © 2001 by The Endocrine Society.

[333] Attallah H, Friedlander AL, Hoffman AR. Visceral obesity, impaired glucose tolerance, metabolic syndrome, and growth hormone therapy. Growth Horm IGF Res. 2006 Jul;16 Suppl A:S62-7.

[334] Franco C; Brandberg J; Lönn L; Andersson B; Bengtsson BA; Johannsson G. Growth hormone treatment reduces abdominal visceral fat in postmenopausal women with abdominal obesity: a 12-month placebo-controlled trial. J Clin Endocrinol Metab. 2005; 90(3):1466-74 (ISSN: 0021-972X)

[335] Colao, A; di Somma, C; et al. Improved Cardiovascular Risk Factors and Cardiac Performance after 12 Months of Growth Hormone (GH) Replacement in Young Adult Patients with GH Deficiency. The Journal of Clinical Endocrinology & Metabolism Vol. 86, No. 5 1874-1881. Copyright © 2001 by The Endocrine Society.

[336] Franco C; Brandberg J; Lönn L; Andersson B; Bengtsson BA; Johannsson G. Growth hormone treatment reduces abdominal visceral fat in postmenopausal women with abdominal obesity: a 12-month placebo-controlled trial. J Clin Endocrinol Metab. 2005; 90(3):1466-74 (ISSN: 0021-972X)

[337] Fukuda I; Hizuka N; Ishikawa Y; Itoh E; Yasumoto K; Murakami Y; Sata A; Tsukada J; Kurimoto M; Okubo Y; Takano K. Serum adiponectin levels in adult growth hormone deficiency and acromegaly. Growth Horm IGF Res. 2004; 14(6):449-54 (ISSN: 1096-6374)

[338] Spina LD, Soares DV, Brasil RR, Lobo PM, Lucia Conceicao F, Vaisman M. Glucose metabolism and visceral fat in GH deficient adults: two years of GH-replacement. Pituitary. 2004;7(3):123-9.

[339] Ramirez RJ, Wolf SE, Barrow RE, Herndon DN. Growth hormone treatment in pediatric burns: a safe therapeutic approach. Ann Surg. 1998 Oct;228(4):439-48.

[340] Mulligan K, Schambelan M. Anabolic treatment with GH, IGF-I, or anabolic steroids in patients with HIV-associated wasting. Int J Cardiol. 2002 Sep;85(1):151-9.

[341] Lange KH ; Lorentsen J ; Isaksson F ; Juul A ; Rasmussen MH ; Christensen NJ ; Bülow J ; Kjaer M. Endurance training and GH administration in elderly women: effects on abdominal adipose tissue lipolysis. Am J Physiol Endocrinol Metab. 2001; 280(6):E886-97 (ISSN: 0193-1849).

[342] O'Connell T; Clemmons DR. IGF-I/IGF-binding protein-3 combination improves insulin resistance by GH-dependent and independent mechanisms. J Clin Endocrinol Metab. 2002; 87(9):4356-60 (ISSN: 0021-972X).

[343] Aberg ND, Brywe KG, Isgaard J. Aspects of growth hormone and insulin-like growth factor-I related to neuroprotection, regeneration, and functional plasticity in the adult brain. ScientificWorldJournal. 2006 Jan 18;6:53-80.

[344] Rezvani I., DiGeorge AM, Dowshen SA, Bourdony CJ. Action of human growth hormone (hGH) on extrathyroidal conversion of thyroxine (T4) to triiodothyronine (T3) in children with hypopituitarism. Pediatric Research, Vol 15, 6-9, Copyright © 1981 by International Pediatric Research Foundation.

[345] Bollerslev J, Hallen J, Fougner KJ, Jorgensen AP, Kristo C, Fagertun H, Gudmundsen O, Burman P, Schreiner T. Low-dose GH improves exercise capacity in adults with GH deficiency: effects of a 22-month placebo-controlled, crossover trial. Eur J Endocrinol. 2005 Sep;153(3):379-87.

[346] Napolitano LA; Lo JC; Gotway MB; Mulligan K; Barbour JD; Schmidt D; Grant RM; Halvorsen RA; Schambelan M; McCune JM. Increased thymic mass and circulating naive CD4 T cells in HIV-1-infected

adults treated with growth hormone. AIDS. 2002; 16(8):1103-11 (ISSN: 0269-9370).

[347] Decker D, Springer W, Tolba R, Lauschke H, Hirner A, von Ruecker A. Perioperative treatment with human growth hormone down-regulates apoptosis and increases superoxide production in PMN from patients undergoing infrarenal abdominal aortic aneurysm repair. Growth Horm IGF Res. 2005 Jun;15(3):193-9.

[348] Van der Lely AJ, Lamberts SW, Jauch KW, Swierstra BA, Hertlein H, Danielle De Vries D, Birkett MA, Bates PC, Blum WF, Attanasio AF. Use of human GH in elderly patients with accidental hip fracture. Eur J Endocrinol. 2000 Nov;143(5):585-92.

[349] Hoffman AR; Kuntze JE; Baptista J; Baum HB; Baumann GP; Biller BM; Clark RV; Cook D; Inzucchi SE; Kleinberg D; Klibanski A; Phillips LS; Ridgway EC; Robbins RJ; Schlechte J; Sharma M; Thorner MO; Vance ML. Growth hormone (GH) replacement therapy in adult-onset gh deficiency: effects on body composition in men and women in a double-blind, randomized, placebo-controlled trial. J Clin Endocrinol Metab. 2004; 89(5):2048-56 (ISSN: 0021-972X).

[350] May Oh, D; Phillips, TJ. Sex Hormones and Wound Healing. Wounds. 2006;18(1):8-18. ©2006 Health Management Publications, Inc

[351] Leal-Cerro A, Povedano J, Astorga R, Gonzalez M, Silva H, Garcia-Pesquera F, Casanueva FF, Dieguez C. The growth hormone (GH)-releasing hormone-GH-insulin-like growth factor-1 axis in patients with fibromyalgia syndrome. J Clin Endocrinol Metab. 1999 Sep;84(9):3378-81.

[352] Hayashi M, Shimohira M, Saisho S, Shimozawa K, Iwakawa Y. Sleep disturbance in children with growth hormone deficiency. Brain Dev. 1992 May;14(3):170-4.

[353] Scheepens A; Sirimanne ES; Breier BH; Clark RG; Gluckman PD; Williams CE. Growth hormone as a neuronal rescue factor during recovery from CNS injury. Neuroscience. 2001; 104(3):677-87 (ISSN: 0306-4522).

[354] Nyberg F. Growth hormone in the brain: characteristics of specific brain targets for the hormone and their functional significance. Front Neuroendocrin. 2000 Oct;21(4):330-48.

[355] Nyberg F. Growth hormone in the brain: characteristics of specific brain targets for the hormone and their functional significance. Front Neuroendocrin. 2000 Oct;21(4):330-48.

[356] Aberg ND, Carlsson B, Rosengren L, Oscarsson J, Isaksson OG, Ronnback L, Eriksson PS. Growth hormone increases connexin-43 expression in the cerebral cortex and hypothalamus. Endocrinology. 2000 Oct;141(10):3879-86.

[357] Sugimoto T, Nakaoka D, Nasu M, Kanzawa M, Sugishita T, Chihara K. Effect of recombinant human growth hormone in elderly osteoporotic women. Clin Endocrinol (Oxf). 1999 Dec;51(6):715-24.

[358] Van der Lely AJ, Lamberts SW, Jauch KW, Swierstra BA, Hertlein H, Danielle De Vries D, Birkett MA, Bates PC, Blum WF, Attanasio AF. Use of human GH in elderly patients with accidental hip fracture. Eur J Endocrinol. 2000 Nov;143(5):585-92.

[359] Rousseau N, Brazeau P, Lapierre H, Abribat T. Effect of aging on growth hormone-induced insulin-like growth factor-I secretion from cultured rat chondrocytes. Growth Horm IGF Res. 1998 Oct;8(5):403-9.

[360] Borson-Chazot F, Serusclat A, Kalfallah Y, Ducottet X, Sassolas G, Bernard S, Labrousse F, Pastene J, Sassolas A, Roux Y, Berthezene F. Decrease in carotid intima-media thickness after one year growth hormone (GH) treatment in adults with GH deficiency. J Clin Endocrinol Metab. 1999 Apr;84(4):1329-33.

[361] Gibney J, Johannsson G. Safety of growth hormone replacement therapy in adults. Expert Opin Drug Saf. 2004 Jul;3(4):305-16.

[362] Sesmilo G, Biller BM, Llevadot J, Hayden D, Hanson G, Rifai N, Klibanski A. Effects of growth hormone administration on inflammatory and other cardiovascular risk markers in men with growth hormone deficiency. A randomized, controlled clinical trial. Ann Intern Med. 2000 Jul 18;133(2):111-22.

[363] Burgess W, Liu Q, Zhou J, Tang Q, Ozawa A, VanHoy R, Arkins S, Dantzer R, Kelley KW. The immune-endocrine loop during aging: role of growth hormone and insulin-like growth factor-I. Neuroimmunomodulation. 1999 Jan-Apr;6(1-2):56-68.

[364] Verhelst, J. et al. Two years of replacement therapy in adults with growth hormone deficiency. Clinical Endocrinology. Volume 47 Page 485 - October 1997 doi:10.1046/j.1365-2265.1997.3041112.x Volume 47 Issue. 4.

[365] Laurie Barclay, MD. Growth Hormone Reduces Weight, Fat Mass But Not Lean Body Mass. Medscape Medical News 2004. © 2004 Medscape. Available online at www.medscape.com/viewarticle/470371.

[366] Van Cauter E, Copinschi G. Interrelationships between growth hormone and sleep. Growth Horm IGF Res. 2000 Apr;10 Suppl B:S57-62.

[367] Laursen, T. Pharmacological aspects of GH Replacement Therapy. Growth Hormone in Adults, 1996, Cambridge University Press.

[368] Winters, SJ. Current Status of Testosterone Replacement Therapy in Men. Arch Fam Med. 1999;8:257-263.

[369] Behre HM. Prostate volume in testosterone-treated and untreated hypogonadal men in comparison to age-matched normal controls. Clin Endocrinol. 1994;40:341-349.

[370] Winters, SJ. Current Status of Testosterone Replacement Therapy in Men. Arch Fam Med. 1999;8:257-263.

[371] A Barqawi; E D Crawford. Testosterone Replacement Therapy and the Risk of Prostate Cancer. Is There a Link? Int J Impot Res. 2006; 18(4):323-328. ©2006 Nature Publishing Group.

[372] Available online at http://www.endo-society.org/quickcontent/clinicalpractice/clinical-guidelines/CG_Androgen.cfm

[373] The Endocrine Society. Testosterone Therapy in Adult Men with Androgen Deficiency Syndromes: An Endocrine Society Clinical Practice Guideline. Available at http://www.endo-society.org/quickcontent/clinicalpractice/clinical-guidelines/CG_Androgen.cfm.

[374] The Endocrine Society. Testosterone Therapy in Adult Men with Androgen Deficiency Syndromes: An Endocrine Society Clinical Practice Guideline. Available at http://www.endo-society.org/quickcontent/clinicalpractice/clinical-guidelines/CG_Androgen.cfm.

[375] Smith AM, Jones RD, Channer KS. The influence of sex hormones on pulmonary vascular reactivity: possible vasodilator therapies for the treatment of pulmonary hypertension. Curr Vasc Pharmacol. 2006 Jan;4(1):9-15.

[376] Golden SH, Maguire A, Ding J, Crouse JR, Cauley JA, Zacur H, Szklo M. Endogenous postmenopausal hormones and carotid atherosclerosis: a case-control study of the atherosclerosis risk in communities cohort. Am J Epidemiol. 2002 Mar 1;155(5):437-45.

[377] Dobrzycki S, Serwatka W, Nadlewski S, et al. An assessment of correlations between endogenous sex hormone levels and the extensiveness of coronary heart disease and the ejection fraction of the left ventricle in males. J Med Invest. 2003 Aug;50(3-4):162-9.

[378] Phillips GB, Pinkernell BH, Jing TY. Are major risk factors for myocardial infarction the major predictors of degree of coronary artery disease in men? Metabolism. 2004 Mar;53(3):324-9.

[379] Dzugan SA, Smith RA. Hypercholesterolemia treatment: a new hypothesis or just an accident? Med Hypothesis. 2002 Dec;59(6):751-6.

[380] Dzugan SA, Smith RA. Broad spectrum restoration in natural steroid hormones as possible treatment for hypercholesterolemia. Bull Urg Rec Med. 2002;3(2):278-84.

[381] English KM, Steeds R, Jones TH, Channer KS: Testosterone and coronary heart disease: is there a link? Q J Med 90:787–791, 1997.

[382] Anderson RA, Ludlam CA, Wu FC: Haemostatic effects of supraphysiological levels of testosterone in normal men. Thromb Haemost 74:693–697, 1995.

[383] Webb CM, McNeill JG, Hayward CS, Zeigler D, Collins P: Effects of testosterone on coronary vasomotor regulation in men with coronary heart disease. Circulation 100:1690–1696, 1999.

[384] Osuna JA, Gomez-Perez R, Arata-Bellabarba G, Villaroel V. Relationship between BMI, total testosterone, sex hormone-binding-globulin, leptin, insulin and insulin resistance in obese men. Arch Androl. 2006 Sep-Oct;52(5):355-61.

[385] Simon D, Charles MA, Nahoul K, Orssaud G, Kremski J, Hully V, Joubert E, Papoz L, Eschwege E: Association between plasma total testosterone and cardiovascular risk factors in healthy adult men: the Telecom
Study. J Clin Endocrinol Metab 82:682–685, 1997.

[386] Abrams D. Use of androgens in patients who have HIV/AIDS: what we know about the effect of androgens on wasting and lipodystrophy. AIDS Read. 2001 Mar;11(3):149-56.

[387] Osuna JA, Gomez-Perez R, Arata-Bellabarba G, Villaroel V. Relationship between BMI, total testosterone, sex hormone-binding-globulin, leptin, insulin and insulin resistance in obese men. Arch Androl. 2006 Sep-Oct;52(5):355-61.

[388] Hogervorst E, Bandelow S, Combrinck M, Smith AD. Low free testosterone is an independent risk factor for Alzheimer's disease. Exp Gerontol. 2004 Nov-Dec;39(11-12):1633-9.

[389] Winters, SJ. Current Status of Testosterone Replacement Therapy in Men. Arch Fam Med. 1999;8:257-

263.

[390] Carrier S, Zvara P, Lue TF. Erectile dysfunction. *Endocrinol Metab Clin North Am.* 1994;23:773-782.

[391] Shifren JL, Braunstein GD, Simon JA, Casson PR, Buster JE, Redmond GP, Burki RE, Ginsburg ES, Rosen RC, Leiblum SR, Caramelli KE, Mazer NA. Transdermal testosterone treatment in women with impaired sexual function after oophorectomy. N Engl J Med. 2000 Sep 7;343(10):682-8.

[392] Mooradian AD, Morley JE, Korenman SG. Biological actions of androgens. *Endocr Rev.* 1987;8:1-28.

[393] Veldhuis JD, Keenan DM, Mielke K, Miles JM, Bowers CY. Testosterone supplementation in healthy older men drives GH and IGF-I secretion without potentiating peptidyl secretagogue efficacy. Eur J Endocrinol. 2005 Oct;153(4):577-86.

[394] Yael Waknine. Testosterone Replacement Improves Exercise Capacity in Men With CHF. [online] Available on Medscape Medical News 2005. © 2005 Medscape at www.medscape.com/viewarticle/506223

[395] Malkin CJ, Pugh PJ, West JN, van Beek EJ, Jones TH, Channer KS. Testosterone therapy in men with moderate severity heart failure: a double-blind randomized placebo controlled trial. Eur Heart J. 2006 Jan;27(1):57-64.

[396] Walston, J; Hadley, EC; Ferrucci, L; Guralnik, JM; Newman, AB; Studenski, SA; Ershler, WB; Harris, T; Fried, LP. Research Agenda for Frailty in Older Adults. J Am Geriatr Soc. 2006;54(6):991-1001. ©2006 Blackwell Publishing.

[397] Hackney AC, Moore AW, Brownlee KK. Testosterone and endurance exercise: development of the "exercise-hypogonadal male condition". Acta Physiol Hung. 2005;92(2):121-37.

[398] Demling RH. The role of anabolic hormones for wound healing in catabolic States. J Burns Wounds. 2005 Jan 17;4:e2.

[399] Hardman MJ, Ashcroft GS. Hormonal influences on wound healing: a review of current experimental data. WOUNDS. 2005;17(11):313-320.

[400] Muller M; Aleman A; Grobbee DE; de Haan EH; van der Schouw YT. Endogenous sex hormone levels and cognitive function in aging men: is there an optimal level? Neurology. 2005; 64(5):866-71 (ISSN: 1526-632X).

[401] Brian C. Lund, Pharm.D., Kristine A. Bever-Stille, Pharm.D., and Paul J. Perry, Ph.D. Testosterone and Andropause: The Feasibility of Testosterone Replacement Therapy in Elderly Men. Pharmacotherapy 19(8):951-956, 1999. © 1999 Pharmacotherapy Publications.

[402] American College of Endocrinologists and American Association of Clinical Endocrinologists. *Guidelines for the Evaluation and Treatment of Male Sexual Dysfunction.* American College of Endocrinologists and American Association of Clinical Endocrinologists; 1998:4.

[403] Aversa A, Isidori AM, De Martino MU, et al. Androgens and penile erection evidence for a direct relationship between free testosterone and cavernous vasodilation in men with ED. Clin Endocrinol (Oxf). 2000;53:517-522.

[404] [Article in Chinese] Chen X, Li X, Huang HY, Li X, Lin JF. [Effects of testosterone on insulin receptor substrate-1 and glucose transporter 4 expression in cells sensitive to insulin] Zhonghua Yi Xue Za Zhi. 2006 Jun 6;86(21):1474-7.

[405] Braga-Basaria M, Dobs AS, Muller DC, Carducci MA, John M, Egan J, Basaria S. Metabolic syndrome in men with prostate cancer undergoing long-term androgen-deprivation therapy. J Clin Oncol. 2006 Aug 20;24(24):3979-83.

[406] Svartberg J. Epidemiology: testosterone and the metabolic syndrome. Int J Impot Res. 2006 Jul 20.

[407] Fogari R, Preti P, Zoppi A, Fogari E, Rinaldi A, Corradi L, Mugellini A. Serum testosterone levels and arterial blood pressure in the elderly. Hypertens Res. 2005 Aug;28(8):625-30.

[408] Huisman HW, Schutte AE, Van Rooyen JM, Malan NT, Malan L, Schutte R, Kruger A. The influence of testosterone on blood pressure and risk factors for cardiovascular disease in a black South African population. Ethn Dis. 2006 Summer;16(3):693-8.

[409] Vondracek, SF; Hansen, LB. Current Approaches to the Management of Osteoporosis in Men. Am J Health-Syst Pharm 61(17):1801-1811, 2004. © 2004 American Society of Health-System Pharmacists.

[410] Isidori AM, Giannetta E, Greco EA, Gianfrilli D, Bonifacio V, Isidori A, Lenzi A, Fabbri A. Effects of testosterone on body composition, bone metabolism and serum lipid profile in middle-aged men: a meta-analysis. Clin Endocrinol (Oxf). 2005 Sep;63(3):280-93.

[411] Reported by By Karla Gale. Testosterone May Slow Progress of MS in Men. Reuters Health Information 2006. © 2006 Reuters Ltd. [online] Available on Medscape® at

www.medscape.com/viewarticle/529199.

[412] Markianos M; Panas M; Kalfakis N; Vassilopoulos D. Plasma testosterone in male patients with Huntington's disease: relations to severity of illness and dementia. Ann Neurol. 2005; 57(4):520-5 (ISSN: 0364-5134).

[413] Moffat SD. Effects of testosterone on cognitive and brain aging in elderly men. Ann N Y Acad Sci. 2005; 1055:80-92 (ISSN: 0077-8923).

[414] Bialek M, Zaremba P, Borowicz KK, Czuczwar SJ. Neuroprotective role of testosterone in the nervous system. Pol J Pharmacol. 2004 Sep-Oct;56(5):509-18.

[415] Finazzi G, Gregg XT, Barbui T, Prchal JT. Idiopathic erythrocytosis and other non-clonal polycythemias. Best Pract Res Clin Haematol. 2006;19(3):471-82.

[416] Ferrucci L, Maggio M, Bandinelli S, Basaria S, Lauretani F, Ble A, Valenti G, Ershler WB, Guralnik JM, Longo DL. Low testosterone levels and the risk of anemia in older men and women. Arch Intern Med. 2006 Jul 10;166(13):1380-8.

[417] McVary KT; McKenna KE. The relationship between erectile dysfunction and lower urinary tract symptoms: epidemiological, clinical, and basic science evidence. Curr Urol Rep. 2004; 5(4):251-7 (ISSN: 1527-2737).

[418] Kaminetsky J. Comorbid LUTS and erectile dysfunction: optimizing their management. Curr Med Res Opin. 2006 Dec;22(12):2497-506.

[419] Spector TD, Perry LA, Tubb G, Silman AJ, Huskisson EC. Low free testosterone levels in rheumatoid arthritis. Ann Rheum Dis. 1988 Jan;47(1):65-8.

[420] Cutolo M, Balleari E, Giusti M, Monachesi M, Accardo S. Sex hormone status of male patients with rheumatoid arthritis: evidence of low serum concentrations of testosterone at baseline and after human chorionic gonadotropin stimulation. Arthritis Rheum. 1988 Oct;31(10):1314-7.

[421] Rhoden EL; Morgentaler A. Testosterone replacement therapy in hypogonadal men at high risk for prostate cancer: results of 1 year of treatment in men with prostatic intraepithelial neoplasia. J Urol. 2003; 170(6 Pt 1):2348-51 (ISSN: 0022-5347)

[422] Smith AM, English KM, Malkin CJ, Jones RD, Jones TH, Channer KS. Testosterone does not adversely affect fibrinogen or tissue plasminogen activator (tPA) and plasminogen activator inhibitor-1 (PAI-1) levels in 46 men with chronic stable angina. Eur J Endocrinol. 2005 Feb;152(2):285-91.

[423] Orwoll E, Lambert LC, Marshall LM, Blank J, Barrett-Connor E, Cauley J, Ensrud K, Cummings SR; Osteoporotic Fractures in Men Study Group. Endogenous testosterone levels, physical performance, and fall risk in older men. Arch Intern Med. 2006 Oct 23;166(19):2124-31.

[424] Winters SJ. Endocrine evaluation of testicular function. *Endocrinol Metab Clin North Am.* 1994;23:709-723.

[425] [no author listed] Available at www.andrologysociety.com/positionstatements. Accessed 2006 Oct 23.

[426] Matsumoto AM, Bremner WJ. Serum testosterone assays—accuracy matters. J. Clin. Endrocrinol.Metab. 2004, 89:520-524.

[427] Stattin P, Soderberg S, Hallmans G, Bylund A, Kaaks R, Stenman UH *et al.* Leptin is associated with increased prostate cancer risk: a nested case-referent study. *J Clin Endocrinol Metab* 2001; 86: 1341-1345.

[428] A Barqawi; E D Crawford. Testosterone Replacement Therapy and the Risk of Prostate Cancer. Is There a Link? Int J Impot Res. 2006; 18(4):323-328. ©2006 Nature Publishing Group.

[429] A diagnosis of polycythemia vera is made when a patent fulfills all three of the major criteria, or any two major and any two minor criteria. Major Criteria: total RBC vol men > 36 mg/kg; women >32 mg/kg ;arterial 02 saturation > 92%; Splenomegaly. Minor Criteria: Platelet count > 400 x 10^9/L; Leukocytosis > 12 x 10^9/L; LAP > 100 (no infection); Serum B12 > 900 pg/ml or UB12 BC> 2200 pg/ml -- Berlin M: Diagnosis and classification of the polycythemias.Semin Hematol 1975; 12:339-341.

[430] Finazzi G, Gregg XT, Barbui T, Prchal JT. Idiopathic erythrocytosis and other non-clonal polycythemias. Best Pract Res Clin Haematol. 2006;19(3):471-82.

[431] Snyder, PJ. What's New in Medicine; Testes and Testicular Disorders. WebMD Scientific American® Medicine 2003. © 2003 WebMD Inc. All rights reserved.[online] Available at www.medscape.com/viewarticle/461007. Accessed 2006 Oct 14.

[432] Zitzmann M, Nieschlag E. Hormone substitution in male hypogonadism. Mol Cell Endocrinol. 2000 Mar 30;161(1-2):73-88.

[433] Finazzi G, Gregg XT, Barbui T, Prchal JT. Idiopathic erythrocytosis and other non-clonal polycythemias. Best Pract Res Clin Haematol. 2006;19(3):471-82.

[434] Margo K; Winn R. Testosterone treatments: why, when, and how? Am Fam Physician. 2006; 73(9):1591-8 (ISSN: 0002-838X).

[435] Ellyin FM. The long term beneficial treatment of low dose testosterone in the aging male. Proc 77th Meeting of The Endocrine Soc., Washington D.C., 1995; 2-127 .

[436] I mamoto T, Suzuki H, Fukasawa S, Shimbo M, Inahara M, Komiya A *et al*. Pretreatment serum testosterone level as a predictive factor of pathological stage in localized prostate cancer patients treated with radical prostatectomy. *Eur Urol* 2005; 47: 308-312.

[437] Massengill JC, Sun L, Moul JW, Wu H, McLeod DG, Amling C *et al*. Pretreatment total testosterone level predicts pathological stage in patients with localized prostate cancer treated with radical prostatectomy. *J Urol* 2003; 169: 1670-1675.

[438] Stattin P, Soderberg S, Hallmans G, Bylund A, Kaaks R, Stenman UH *et al*. Leptin is associated with increased prostate cancer risk: a nested case-referent study. *J Clin Endocrinol Metab* 2001; 86: 1341-1345.

[439] Melmed, S. Endocrinology, Pituitary: Anterior Pituitary Hormones and Associated Disorders. ACP Medicine Online. 2002; ©2002 WebMD Inc. Available at www.medscape.com/viewarticle/535179. Accessed 2006 Oct 14.

[440] Presti J, McNeal J, Hsu T, Brooks J, Gill H. Performance of PSA levels between 4 and 10 ng/mL in the era of extended biopsy schemes. Program and abstracts of the American Urological Association 2006 Annual Meeting; May 20-25, 2006; Atlanta, Georgia. Abstract 468.

[441] Stamey TA, Caldwell M, McNeal JE, Nolley R, Hemenez M, Downs J. The prostate specific antigen era in the United States is over for prostate cancer: what happened in the last 20 years? J Urol. 2004;172:1297-1301.

[442] [no author listed] QuickStats: Percentage of Men Aged >40 Years* with Prostate-Specific Antigen Levels of >2.5 and >4.0 ng/mL by Race/Ethnicity — National Health and Nutrition Examination Survey, United States, 2001-2004. MMWR. 2006;55(48):1305. ©2006 Centers for Disease Control and Prevention (CDC).

[443] Andrews RC; Herlihy O; Livingstone DE; Andrew R; Walker BR. Abnormal cortisol metabolism and tissue sensitivity to cortisol in patients with glucose intolerance. J Clin Endocrinol Metab. 2002; 87(12):5587-93 (ISSN: 0021-972X).

[444] Andrews RC; Herlihy O; Livingstone DE; Andrew R; Walker BR. Abnormal cortisol metabolism and tissue sensitivity to cortisol in patients with glucose intolerance. J Clin Endocrinol Metab. 2002; 87(12):5587-93 (ISSN: 0021-972X).

[445] Neki NS; Singh RB; Rastogi SS. How brain influences neuro-cardiovascular dysfunction. J Assoc Physicians India. 2004; 52:223-30 (ISSN: 0004-5772).

[446] O'Connor, PG. Psychiatry: Alcohol Abuse and Dependency: Common Problems Associated with Alcohol Abuse. ACP Medicine Online. 2002; ©2002 WebMD Inc. [online] Available at www.medscape.com/viewarticle/534449. Accessed 2006 Oct 14.

[447] Falch JA, Steihaug S. Vitamin D deficiency in Pakistani premenopausal women living in Norway is not associated with evidence of reduced skeletal strength. Scand J Clin Lab Invest. 2000 Apr;60(2):103-9.

[448] Theiler R, Stahelin HB, Kranzlin M, Somorjai G, Singer-Lindpaintner L, Conzelmann M, Geusens P, Bischoff HA. Influence of physical mobility and season on 25-hydroxyvitamin D-parathyroid hormone interaction and bone remodelling in the elderly. Eur J Endocrinol. 2000 Nov;143(5):673-9.

[449] Kapoor M, Chan GZ. Fluid and electrolyte abnormalities. Crit Care Clin 2001;17:503-29.

[450] [no authors listed][online] http://en.wikipedia.org/wiki/Chvostek's_sign. Accessed March 27, 2007.

[451] [no authors listed][online] http://en.wikipedia.org/wiki/Trousseau_sign_of_latent_tetany. Accessed March 27, 2007.

[452] Holick MF. Vitamin D: photobiology, metabolism, mechanism of action, and clinical applications. In: Favus MJ, ed. Primer on the metabolic bone diseases and disorders of mineral metabolism. 5th ed. Washington, D.C.: American Society for Bone and Mineral Research, 2003;129-37.

[453] Yew KS, DeMieri PJ. Disorders of bone mineral metabolism. Clin Fam Pract 2002;4:525-65.

[454] Masuyama R, Stockmans I, Torrekens S, Van Looveren R, Maes C, Carmeliet P, Bouillon R, Carmeliet G. Vitamin D receptor in chondrocytes promotes osteoclastogenesis and regulates FGF23 production in osteoblasts. J Clin Invest. 2006 Dec;116(12):3150-9.

[455] Zittermann A, Schleithoff SS, Koerfer R. Vitamin D insufficiency in congestive heart failure: why and what to do about it? Heart Fail Rev. 2006 Mar;11(1):25-33.

[456] Luong KV, Nguyen LT. Vitamin D and cardiovascular disease. Curr Med Chem. 2006;13(20):2443-7.

[457] Tangpricha V, Turner A, Spina C, Decastro S, Chen TC, Holick MF. Tanning is associated with optimal vitamin D status (serum 25-hydroxyvitamin D concentration) and higher bone mineral density. Am J Clin Nutr 2004;80:1645–9.

[458] Zittermann A, Schleithoff SS, Koerfer R. Putting cardiovascular disease and vitamin D insufficiency into perspective. Br J Nutr. 2005 Oct;94(4):483-92.

[459] Luong KV, Nguyen LT. Vitamin D and cardiovascular disease. Curr Med Chem. 2006;13(20):2443-7.

[460] Bischoff HA, Stahelin HB, Dick W, et al. Effects of vitamin D and calcium supplementation on falls: a randomized controlled trial. J Bone Miner Res. 2003 Feb;18(2):343-51.

[461] Kirn, TF. Vitamin D Lowered Risk of Falling in Nursing Homes by 49%. Family Practice News. Volume 31, Issue 24, Page 6 (15 December 2001).

[462] Bischoff-Ferrari HA, Orav EJ, Dawson-Hughes B. Effect of cholecalciferol plus calcium on falling in ambulatory older men and women: a 3-year randomized controlled trial. Arch Intern Med. 2006 Feb 27;166(4):424-30.

[463] Kirn, TF. Vitamin D Lowered Risk of Falling in Nursing Homes by 49%. Family Practice News. Volume 31, Issue 24, Page 6 (15 December 2001).

[464] Bischoff-Ferrari HA, Orav EJ, Dawson-Hughes B. Effect of cholecalciferol plus calcium on falling in ambulatory older men and women: a 3-year randomized controlled trial. Arch Intern Med. 2006 Feb 27;166(4):424-30.

[465] Visser, M., Deeg, D. J., Puts, M. T., Seidell, J. C, Lips, P. (2006). Low serum concentrations of 25-hydroxyvitamin D in older persons and the risk of nursing home admission.. *Am. J. Clin. Nutr.* 84: 616-622.

[466] Colston KW, Lowe LC, Mansi JL, Campbell MJ. Vitamin D status and breast cancer risk. Anticancer Res. 2006 Jul-Aug;26(4A):2573-80.

[467] Bertone-Johnson ER, Chen WY, Holick MF, Hollis BW, Colditz GA, Willett WC, Hankinson SE. Plasma 25-hydroxyvitamin D and 1,25-dihydroxyvitamin D and risk of breast cancer. Cancer Epidemiol Biomarkers Prev. 2005 Aug;14(8):1991-7.

[468] Feskanich D, Ma J, Fuchs CS, *et al.* Plasma vitamin D metabolites and risk of colorectal cancer in women. Cancer Epidemiol Biomarkers Prev 2004; 13:1502-1508.
* This was the largest study to show an inverse association between 25(OH)D level and colorectal cancer risk.

[469] Garland CF, Mohr SB, Gorham ED,   Grant WB, Garland FC. Role of ultraviolet B irradiance and vitamin D in prevention of ovarian cancer. Am J Prev Med. 2006 Dec;31(6):512-4.

[470] Skinner HG, Michaud DS, Giovannucci E, Willett WC, Colditz GA, Fuchs CS. Vitamin D intake and the risk for pancreatic cancer in two cohort studies. Cancer Epidemiol Biomarkers Prev. 2006 Sep;15(9):1688-95.

[471] Munger KL, Levin LI, Hollis BW, Howard NS, Ascherio A. Serum 25-hydroxyvitamin D levels and risk of multiple sclerosis. JAMA. 2006 Dec 20;296(23):2832-8.

[472] Banerjee TK, Mukherjee A, Bhargava A. Childhood multiple sclerosis--report of two Indian cases. J Assoc Physicians India. 2002 Aug;50:1091-2.

[473] Thomas, K.M., Lloyd-Jones, D.M., et al. Hypovitaminosis D in Medical Inpatients. NEJM. March 19, 1998. Volume 338:777-783.

[474] Kamen DL, Cooper GS, Bouali H, Shaftman SR, Hollis BW, Gilkeson GS. Vitamin D deficiency in systemic lupus erythematosus. Autoimmun Rev. 2006 Feb;5(2):114-7.

[475] Dealberto MJ. Why are immigrants at increased risk for psychosis? Vitamin D insufficiency, epigenetic mechanisms, or both? Med Hypotheses. 2007;68(2):259-67.

[476] Zittermann A, Schleithoff SS, Koerfer R. Vitamin D insufficiency in congestive heart failure: why and what to do about it? Heart Fail Rev. 2006 Mar;11(1):25-33.

[477] Bischof MG, Heinze G, Vierhapper H. Vitamin D status and its relation to age and body mass index. Horm Res. 2006;66(5):211-5.

[478] Al-Allaf AW, Mole PA, Paterson CR, Pullar T. Bone health in patients with fibromyalgia. Rheumatology (Oxford). 2003 Oct;42(10):1202-6.

[479] Vieth R; Bischoff-Ferrari H; Boucher BJ; Dawson-Hughes B; Garland CF; Heaney RP; Holick MF; Hollis BW; Lamberg-Allardt C; McGrath JJ; Norman AW; Scragg R; Whiting SJ; Willett WC; Zittermann A. The urgent need to recommend an intake of vitamin D that is effective. Am J Clin Nutr. 2007;

85(3):649-50 (ISSN: 0002-9165).

[480] Armas LA, Hollis BW, Heaney RP. Vitamin D2 is much less effective than vitamin D3 in humans. J Clin Endocrinol Metab. 2004 Nov;89(11):5387-91.

[481] Calvo MS, Whiting SJ, Barton CN. Vitamin D intake: a global perspective of current status. J Nutr. 2005 Feb;135(2):310-6.

[482] R. Vieth, H. Bischoff-Ferrari, B. J Boucher, B. Dawson-Hughes, C. F Garland, R. P Heaney, M. F Holick, B. W Hollis, C. Lamberg-Allardt, J. J McGrath, A. W Norman, R. Scragg, S. J Whiting, W. C Willett, and A. Zittermann. The urgent need to recommend an intake of vitamin D that is effective. Am. J. Clinical Nutrition, March 1, 2007; 85(3): 649 - 650.

[483] R. Vieth, H. Bischoff-Ferrari, B. J Boucher, B. Dawson-Hughes, C. F Garland, R. P Heaney, M. F Holick, B. W Hollis, C. Lamberg-Allardt, J. J McGrath, A. W Norman, R. Scragg, S. J Whiting, W. C Willett, and A. Zittermann. The urgent need to recommend an intake of vitamin D that is effective. Am. J. Clinical Nutrition, March 1, 2007; 85(3): 649 - 650.

[484] Vieth R; Bischoff-Ferrari H; Boucher BJ; Dawson-Hughes B; Garland CF; Heaney RP; Holick MF; Hollis BW; Lamberg-Allardt C; McGrath JJ; Norman AW; Scragg R; Whiting SJ; Willett WC; Zittermann A. The urgent need to recommend an intake of vitamin D that is effective. Am J Clin Nutr. 2007; 85(3):649-50 (ISSN: 0002-9165).

[485] J. Endocrinol. Invest. 2004;27:807–12

[486] Campbell B, Roberts M, Kerksick C, Wilborn C, Marcello B, Taylor L, Nassar E, Leutholtz B, Bowden R, Rasmussen C, Greenwood M, Kreider R. Pharmacokinetics, safety, and effects on exercise performance of l-arginine alpha-ketoglutarate in trained adult men. Nutrition. 2006 Sep;22(9):872-81.

[487] Miller AL. The effects of sustained-release-L-arginine formulation on blood pressure and vascular compliance in 29 healthy individuals. Altern Med Rev. 2006 Mar;11(1):23-9.

[488] Yang EH, Barsness GW. Evolving.treatment strategies for chronic refractory angina. Expert Opin Pharmacother. 2006 Feb;7(3):259-66.

[489] Hayashi T, Esaki T, Sumi D, Mukherjee T, Iguchi A, Chaudhuri G. Modulating role of estradiol on arginase II expression in hyperlipidemic rabbits as an atheroprotective mechanism. Proc Natl Acad Sci U S A. 2006 Jul 5;103(27):10485-90.

[490] Miller AL. The effects of sustained-release-L-arginine formulation on blood pressure and vascular compliance in 29 healthy individuals. Altern Med Rev. 2006 Mar;11(1):23-9.

[491] Schlaich MP, Oehmer S, Schneider MP, Delles C, Schmidt BM, Schmieder RE. Effects of nitric oxide synthase inhibition and l-arginine on renal haemodynamics in young patients at high cardiovascular risk. Atherosclerosis. 2006 Jun 7.

[492] Aydin S, Inci O, Alagol B. The role of arginine, indomethacin and kallikrein in the treatment of oligoasthenospermia. Int Urol Nephrol. 1995;27(2):199-202.

[493] Doutreleau S, Mettauer B, Piquard F, Rouyer O, Schaefer A, Lonsdorfer J, Geny B. Chronic L-arginine supplementation enhances endurance exercise tolerance in heart failure patients. Int J Sports Med. 2006 Jul;27(7):567-72.

[494] Izhar U, Schwalb H, Borman JB, Merin G. Cardioprotective effect of L-arginine in myocardial ischemia and reperfusion in an isolated working rat heart model. J Cardiovasc Surg (Torino). 1998 Jun;39(3):321-9.

[495] Srivastava S, Desai P, Coutinho E, Govil G. Mechanism of action of L-arginine on the vitality of spermatozoa is primarily through increased biosynthesis of nitric oxide. Biol Reprod. 2006 May;74(5):954-8.

[496] Nagasaka H, Yorifuji T, Murayama K, Kubota M, Kurokawa K, Murakami T, Kanazawa M, Takatani T, Ogawa A, Ogawa E, Yamamoto S, Adachi M, Kobayashi K, Takayanagi M. Effects of arginine treatment on nutrition, growth and urea cycle function in seven Japanese boys with late-onset ornithine transcarbamylase deficiency. Eur J Pediatr. 2006 Sep;165(9):618-24.

[497] Thal LJ, Calvani M, Amato A, Carta A. A 1-year controlled trial of acetyl-l-carnitine in early-onset AD. Neurology. 2000 Sep 26;55(6):805-10

[498] Cooper R, Morre DJ, Morre DM. Medicinal benefits of green tea: Part I. Review of noncancer health benefits. J Altern Complement Med. 2005 Jun;11(3):521-8.

[499] Marwick C. Survey says patients expect little physician help on sex. JAMA. 1999;281:2173-2174.

[500] Lewis RW, Fugl-Meyer KS, Bosch R, Fugl-Meyer AR, Laumann EO, Lizza E, Martin-Morales A. Epidemiology/risk factors of sexual dysfunction. J Sex Med. 2004 Jul;1(1):35-9.

[501] D. Kapoor; C. J. Malkin; K. S. Channer; T. H. Jones. Androgens, Insulin Resistance and Vascular Disease in Men. Clin Endocrinol. 2005;63(3):239-250. ©2005 Blackwell Publishing.

[502] Jonides, LK. National Association of Pediatric Nurse Practitioners (NAPNAP) 25th Annual Conference Highlights of the National Association of Pediatric Nurse Practitioners (NAPNAP) 25th Annual Conference on Pediatric Healthcare. What Children Are Eating: For Many -- It's Too Much! [online] Available at http://www.medscape.com/viewarticle/474963. Accessed 2006 Aug 7.

[503] [no author listed] Obesity and overweight. [online] Available at www.who.int/dietphysicalactivity/publications/facts/obesity/en. Accessed 2006 Aug 7.

[504] Balady GJ, Larson MG, et al. Usefulness of exercise testing in the prediction of coronary disease risk among asymptomatic persons as a function of the Framingham risk score. Circulation. 2004 Oct 5;110(14):1920-5. Epub 2004 Sep 27. . [online] Available at www.ncbi.nlm.nih.gov/entrez/query.fcgi?cmd=Retrieve&db=pubmed&dopt=Abstract&list_uids=15451778&query_hl=11&itool=pubmed_docsum. Accessed 2006 Aug 6.

[505] Wattanakit, K; Folsom, A; et al. Risk Factors for Cardiovascular Event Recurrence in the Atherosclerosis Risk in Communities (ARIC) Study. Am Heart J. 2005; 149 (4): 606-612. ©2005 Mosby, Inc.

[506] Naghavi M, Falk E, Hecht HS, Jamieson MJ, Kaul S, Berman D, Fayad Z, Budoff MJ, Rumberger J, Naqvi TZ, Shaw LJ, Faergeman O, Cohn J, Bahr R, Koenig W, Demirovic J, Arking D, Herrera VL, Badimon J, Goldstein JA, Rudy Y, Airaksinen J, Schwartz RS, Riley WA, Mendes RA, Douglas P, Shah PK; SHAPE Task Force. From vulnerable plaque to vulnerable patient--Part III: Executive summary of the Screening for Heart Attack Prevention and Education (SHAPE) Task Force report. Am J Cardiol. 2006 Jul 17;98(2A):2H-15H.

[507] Pugliese F, Mollet NR, Nieman K, et al. Sixty-four slice CT improves diagnostic accuracy in the detection of coronary artery stenosis in vessels < 2 mm diameter. Program and abstracts of the Radiological Society of North America 91st Scientific Assembly and Annual Meeting; November 27-December 2, 2005; Chicago, Illinois. Page 191.

[508] Johnson, TRC; Nikolaou, K; et al. ECG-Gated 64-MDCT Angiography in the Differential Diagnosis of Acute Chest Pain. Am J Roentgenol. 2007;188(1):76-82. ©2007 American Roentgen Ray Society.

[509] Blair SN, Kohl HW 3rd, Paffenbarger RS Jr, Clark DG, Cooper KH, Gibbons LW. Institute for Aerobics Research, Dallas, Tex 75230. Physical fitness and all-cause mortality. A prospective study of healthy men and women. JAMA. 1989 Nov 3;262(17):2395-401.

[510] Exercise Capacity Predicts Longevity Myers, J., Prakash, M., Froelicher, V., Do, D., Partington, S., and Atwood, J.E. Exercise Capacity and Mortality among Men Referred for Exercise Testing. NEJM; Volume 346:793-801 March 14, 2002. Number 11.

[511] Molly B. Conroy; Nancy R. Cook; Joann E. Manson; Julie E. Buring; I-Min Lee. Past Physical Activity, Current Physical Activity, and the Risk of Coronary Heart Disease. Med Sci Sports Exerc. 2005;37(8):1251-1256. ©2005 American College of Sports Medicine.

[512] Laurie Barclay, MD. New IOM Diet and Exercise Guidelines: A Newsmaker Interview With Joanne R. Lupton, PhD. Available online at www.medscape.com/viewarticle/441639. Accessed 2006 Oct 4.

[513] Sesso HD, Paffenbarger RS Jr, Lee IM. Physical activity and coronary heart disease in men: The Harvard Alumni Health Study. Circulation. 2000 Aug 29;102(9):975-80.

[514] Gregg EW, Gerzoff RB, Caspersen CJ, Williamson DF, Narayan KM. Relationship of walking to mortality among US adults with diabetes. Arch Intern Med. 2003 Jun 23;163(12):1440-7.

[515] Hu FB, Stamfer MJ, Colditz GA, Ascherio A., Rexrode KM, Willet WC, et al. Physical activity and risk of stroke in women. JAMA 2000; 283: 2961-67.

[516] Murphy MH, Hardman AE. Training effects of short and long bouts of brisk walking in sedentary women. Med Sci Sports Exerc. 1998 Jan;30(1):152-7.

[517] Manson JE, Hu FB, Rich-Edwards JW, Colditz GA, Stampfer MJ, Speizer FE, Willett WC, Hennekens CH. A prospective study of walking as compared with vigorous exercise in the prevention of coronary heart disease in women. N Engl J Med. 1999 Aug 26;341(9):650-8.

[518] Jeon CY, Lokken RP, Hu FB, van Dam RM. Physical activity of moderate intensity and risk of type 2 diabetes: a systematic review. Diabetes Care. 2007 Mar;30(3):744-52.

[519] Lee MR, Kim WS. The effects of brisk walking versus brisk walking plus diet on triglycerides and apolipoprotein B levels in middle-aged overweight/obese women with high triglyceride levels. Taehan Kanho Hakhoe Chi. 2006 Dec;36(8):1352-8.

[520] [online] Available at www.shapeup.org/10000steps.html. Accessed March 23, 2007.

[521] Rodier, H. Practical Principles of Advising Patients on Nutrition. Utah Medical Association Bulletin. Vol. 52, No. 11-12;6-7. Nov-Dec 2005.

[522] J. Proceedings of the National Academy of Science, November 12th, 2002.

[523] Peppa M, Uribarri J, Vlassara H. Glucose, advanced glycation end products, and diabetes complications: what is new and what works. Journal of Clinical Diabetes. 2003;21:186-7.

[524] Goldberg T, Cai W, Peppa M, Dardaine V, Baliga BS, Uribarri J, Vlassara H. Advanced glycoxidation end products in commonly consumed foods. J Am Diet Assoc. 2004 Aug;104(8):1287-91.

[525] Taubes, G. "The Soft Science of Dietary Fat," J. Science. 2001;291:2536.

[526] Hwang, G; Lee, D. Trans-fat: The latest and worst fat on the block. J. Family Practice Recertification, Feb. 2005;(27)2:49.

[527] [no author listed] Thought for food Lancet. 2003 Nov 15;362(9396):1593.

[528] Food Politics: How the food industry influences nutrition and health, Marion Nestle, MD, 2003.

[529] Fields, S. Environews, Spheres of Influence, The Fat of the Land: Do Agricultural Subsidies Foster Poor Health? Environ Health Perspect. 2004 October; 112(14): A820–A823.

[530] Korner J, Leibel RL. To eat or not to eat - how the gut talks to the brain. N Engl J Med. 2003 Sep 4;349(10):926-8.

[531] Heim C, Newport DJ, Heit S, Graham YP, Wilcox M, Bonsall R, Miller AH, Nemeroff CB. Pituitary-adrenal and autonomic responses to stress in women after sexual and physical abuse in childhood. JAMA. 2000 Aug 2;284(5):592-7.

[532] Self-efficacy: The Exercise of Control, Albert Bandura, 1997- NewYork: Freeman.

[533] Comparison of the Atkins, Ornish, Weight Watchers, and Zone Diets for Weight Loss and Heart Disease Risk Reduction. A Randomized Trial Michael L. Dansinger, MD; Joi Augustin Gleason, MS, RD; John L. Griffith, PhD; Harry P. Selker, MD, MSPH; Ernst J. Schaefer, MD JAMA. 2005;293:43-53.

[534] Eckel RH. The dietary approach to obesity: is it the diet or the disorder? JAMA. 2005; 293(1):96-7 (ISSN: 1538-3598).

[535] Ello-Martin JA; Ledikwe JH; Rolls BJ. The influence of food portion size and energy density on energy intake: implications for weight management. Am J Clin Nutr. 2005; 82(1 Suppl):236S-241S (ISSN: 0002-9165).

[536] Esposito K, Marfella R, Ciotola M, Di Palo C, Giugliano F, Giugliano G, D'Armiento M, D'Andrea F, Giugliano D. Effect of a mediterranean-style diet on endothelial dysfunction and markers of vascular inflammation in the metabolic syndrome: a randomized trial. JAMA. 2004 Sep 22;292(12):1440-6.

[537] Holly R. Wyatt, Gary K. Grunwald, Cecilia L. Mosca, University of Colorado Health Sciences Center, Denver, CO; Mary L. Klem, University of Pittsburgh School of Medicine, Pittsburgh, PA; Rena R. Wing, Brown Medical School, Providence, RI; James O. Hill, Univeristy of Colorado Health Sciences Center, Denver, CO. Long-termWeight Loss and Breakfast Consumption in Reduced-Obese Subjects in the National Weight Control Registry. AJCN 2002;75supp:365.

[538] Rendell M. Dietary treatment of diabetes mellitus. N Engl J Med. 2000 May 11;342(19):1440-1.

[539] Weigle, DS; Breen, PA; et al. A high-protein diet induces sustained reductions in appetite, ad libitum caloric intake, and body weight despite compensatory changes in diurnal plasma leptin and ghrelin concentrations. Am J Clin Nutr 2005 82: 41-48.

[540] Available online at http://www.hugorodier.com. We highly advise going to visit his website – he is not associated in any way with Program 120® but we think he's very forward thinking.

[541] Gibney, MJ; Walsh, M; Brennan, L; Roche, HM; German, B: van Ommen, B. Metabolomics in human nutrition: opportunities and challenges. Am J Clin Nutr 2005 82: 497-503.

[542] Pawlow LA; O'Neil PM; Malcolm RJ. Night eating syndrome: effects of brief relaxation training on stress, mood, hunger, and eating patterns. Int J Obes Relat Metab Disord. 2003; 27(8):970-8 (ISSN: 0307-0565).

[543] Balsiger BM, Murr MM, Poggio JL, Sarr MG. Bariatric surgery. Surgery for weight control in patients

with morbid obesity. Med Clin North Am. 2000;84:477-489.

[544] Virji A, Murr MM. Caring for patients after bariatric surgery. Am Fam Physician. 2006 Apr 15;73(8):1403-8.

[545] Gastrointestinal surgery for severe obesity. Consens Statement 1991;9:1-20. Accessed online Msrch 26, 2007, at: http://consensus.nih.gov/1991/1991GISurgeryObesity084html.htm.

[546] Pandolfino, JE; Krishnamoorthy, B; Lee, TJ. MedGenMed Gastroenterology. Gastrointestinal Complications of Obesity Surgery. Medscape General Medicine. 2004;6(2):15. ©2004 Medscape. Available at www.medscape.com/viewarticle/471952. Accessed 2006 Aug 9.

[547] Buchwald H, Avidor Y, Braunwald E, Jensen MD, Pories W, Fahrbach K, et al. Bariatric surgery: a systematic review and meta-analysis [published correction appears in JAMA 2005;293:1728]. JAMA 2004;292:1724-37.

[548] Balsiger BM, Kennedy FP, Abu-Lebdeh HS, Collazo-Clavell M, Jensen MD, O'Brien T, et al. Prospective evaluation of Roux-en-Y bypass as primary operation for medically complicated obesity. Mayo Clin Proc 2000;75:673-80.

[549] Virji A, Murr MM. Caring for patients after bariatric surgery. Am Fam Physician. 2006 Apr 15;73(8):1403-8.

[550] Buchwald H, Avidor Y, Braunwald E, Jensen MD, Pories W, Fahrbach K, et al. Bariatric surgery: a systematic review and meta-analysis [published correction appears in JAMA 2005;293:1728]. JAMA 2004;292:1724-37.

[551] Buchwald H, Avidor Y, Braunwald E, Jensen MD, Pories W, Fahrbach K, et al. Bariatric surgery: a systematic review and meta-analysis [published correction appears in JAMA 2005;293:1728]. JAMA 2004;292:1724-37.

[552] Virji A, Murr MM. Caring for patients after bariatric surgery. Am Fam Physician. 2006 Apr 15;73(8):1403-8.

[553] Harper J, Madan AK, Ternovits CA, Tichansky DS. What happens to patients who do not follow-up after bariatric surgery? Am Surg. 2007 Feb;73(2):181-4

[554] Mason EE. Voluntary or obligatory? IBSR Newsletter Summer 2003, vol. 18. Accessed online March 27, 2007, at: http://www.healthcare.uiowa.edu/surgery/ibsr/wsummer03.htm

[555] Sapala JA, Wood MH, Schuhknecht MP, Sapala MA. Fatal pulmonary embolism after bariatric operations for morbid obesity: a 24-year retrospective analysis. Obes Surg 2003;13:819-25.

[556] Virji A, Murr MM. Caring for patients after bariatric surgery. Am Fam Physician. 2006 Apr 15;73(8):1403-8.

[557] Flum DR, Dellinger EP. Impact of gastric bypass operation on survival: a population-based analysis. J Am Coll Surg. 2004 Oct;199(4):543-51.

[558] Virji A, Murr MM. Caring for patients after bariatric surgery. Am Fam Physician. 2006 Apr 15;73(8):1403-8.

[559] Christou NV, Jarand J, Sylvestre JL, McLean AP. Analysis of the incidence and risk factors for wound infections in open bariatric surgery. Obes Surg 2004;14:16-22.

[560] Podnos YD, Jimenez JC, Wilson SE, Stevens CM, Nguyen NT. Complications after laparoscopic gastric bypass: a review of 3464 cases. Arch Surg 2004;138:957-61.

[561] Harper J, Madan AK, Ternovits CA, Tichansky DS. What happens to patients who do not follow-up after bariatric surgery? Am Surg. 2007 Feb;73(2):181-4.

[562] Harper J, Madan AK, Ternovits CA, Tichansky DS. What happens to patients who do not follow-up after bariatric surgery? Am Surg. 2007 Feb;73(2):181-4.

[563] Gohil BC, Sacks BC, McCloskey C, Eid GM, Ramanathan RC. Intussusception following laparoscopic Roux-en-Y gastric bypass surgery for morbid obesity. SOARD 2:386, 2006 (abstract from the IBSR Newsletter Summer 2006. Accessed online March 27, 2007, at: http://www.healthcare.uiowa.edu/surgery/ibsr/wsummer06.htm).

[564] Iglezias Brandao de Oliveira C, Adami Chaim E, Borges da Silva B. Impact of rapid weight reduction on risk of cholelithiasis after bariatric surgery. Obes Surg 2003;13:625-8.

[565] Balsinger BM, Murr MM, Poggio JL, Sarr MG. Bariatric surgery. Surgery for weight control in patients with morbid obesity. Med Clin North Am 2000;84:477-89.

[566] Virji A, Murr MM. Caring for patients after bariatric surgery. Am Fam Physician. 2006 Apr 15;73(8):1403-8.

[567] Bohn M, Way M, Jamieson A. The effect of practical dietary counseling on food variety and

regurgitation frequency after gastroplasty for obesity. Obes Surg 1993;3:23-8.

[568] Virji A, Murr MM. Caring for patients after bariatric surgery. Am Fam Physician. 2006 Apr 15;73(8):1403-8.

[569] McMahon MM; Sarr MG; Clark MM; Gall MM; Knoetgen J; Service FJ; Laskowski ER; Hurley DL. Clinical management after bariatric surgery: value of a multidisciplinary approach. Mayo Clin Proc. 2006; 81(10 Suppl):S34-45 (ISSN: 0025-6196).

[570] Virji A, Murr MM. Caring for patients after bariatric surgery. Am Fam Physician. 2006 Apr 15;73(8):1403-8.

[571] Schauer PR, Ikramuddin S, Gourash W, Ramanathan R, Luketich J. Outcomes after laparoscopic Roux-en-Y gastric bypass for morbid obesity. Ann Surg. 2000;232:515-529.

Made in the USA
Lexington, KY
30 March 2019